Thyroid and Parathyroid Glands: Imaging, Treatment, and Beyond

Guest Editor

LAURIE A. LOEVNER, MD

CLINICS IN NEUROIMAGING

www.neuroimaging.theclinics.com

Consulting Editor

SURESH K. MUKHERJI, MD

August 2008 • Volume 18 • Number 3

SAUNDERS an imprint of ELSEVIER, Inc.

W.B. SAUNDERS COMPANY
A Division of Elsevier Inc.

1600 John F. Kennedy Boulevard • Suite 1800 • Philadelphia, Pennsylvania 19103-2899

http://www.theclinics.com

NEUROIMAGING CLINICS Volume 18, Number 3
August 2008 ISSN 1052-5149, ISBN 13: 978-1-4160-6320-9, ISBN 10: 1-4160-6320-X

Editor: Lisa Richman

© **2008 Elsevier** ■ **All rights reserved.**

This journal and the individual contributions contained in it are protected under copyright by Elsevier, and the following terms and conditions apply to their use:

Photocopying

Single photocopies of single articles may be made for personal use as allowed by national copyright laws. Permission of the Publisher and payment of a fee is required for all other photocopying, including multiple or systematic copying, copying for advertising or promotional purposes, resale, and all forms of document delivery. Special rates are available for educational institutions that wish to make photocopies for non-profit educational classroom use. For information on how to seek permission visit www.elsevier.com/permissions or call: (+44) 1865 843830 (UK)/ (+1) 215 239 3804 (USA).

Derivative Works

Subscribers may reproduce tables of contents or prepare lists of articles including abstracts for internal circulation within their institutions. Permission of the Publisher is required for resale or distribution outside the institution. Permission of the Publisher is required for all other derivative works, including compilations and translations (please consult www.elsevier.com/permissions).

Electronic Storage or Usage

Permission of the Publisher is required to store or use electronically any material contained in this journal, including any article or part of an article (please consult www.elsevier.com/permissions). Except as outlined above, no part of this publication may be reproduced, stored in a retrieval system or transmitted in any form or by any means, electronic, mechanical, photocopying, recording or otherwise, without prior written permission of the Publisher.

Notice

No responsibility is assumed by the Publisher for any injury and/or damage to persons or property as a matter of products liability, negligence or otherwise, or from any use or operation of any methods, products, instructions or ideas contained in the material herein. Because of rapid advances in the medical sciences, in particular, independent verification of diagnoses and drug dosages should be made. Although all advertising material is expected to conform to ethical (medical) standards, inclusion in this publication does not constitute a guarantee or endorsement of the quality or value of such product or of the claims made of it by its manufacturer.

Neuroimaging Clinics (ISSN 1052-5149) is published quarterly by Elsevier Inc., 360 Park Avenue South, New York, NY 10010-1710. Months of issue are February, May, August, and November. Business and editorial offices: 1600 John F. Kennedy Blvd., Suite 1800, Philadelphia, PA 19103-2899. Business and editorial offices: 6277 Sea Harbor Drive, Orlando, FL 32887-4800. Periodicals postage paid at New York, NY, and additional mailing offices. Subscription prices are USD 240 per year for US individuals, USD 370 per year for US institutions, USD 123 per year for US students and residents, USD 277 per year for Canadian individuals, USD 454 per year for Canadian institutions, USD 332 per year for international individuals, USD 454 per year for international institutions and USD 166 per year for Canadian and foreign students and residents. To receive student/resident rate, orders must be accompanied by name of affiliated institution, date of term, and the *signature* of program/residency coordinator on institution letterhead. Orders will be billed at individual rate until proof of status is received. Foreign air speed delivery is included in all *Clinics* subscription prices. All prices are subject to change without notice. POSTMASTER: Send address changes to *Neuroimaging Clinics*, Elsevier Periodicals Customer Service, 6277 Sea Harbor Drive, Orlando, FL 32887-4800. **Customer Service: 1-800-654-2452 (US). From outside the United States, call 1-407-563-6020. Fax: 1-407-363-9661. E-mail: JournalsCustomerService-usa@elsevier.com.**

Reprints. For copies of 100 or more of articles in this publication, please contact the Commercial Reprints Department, Elsevier Inc., 360 Park Avenue South, New York, NY 10010-1710. Tel.: 212-633-3812; Fax: 212-462-1935; E-mail: reprints@elsevier.com.

Neuroimaging Clinics is covered by *Excerpta Medical/EMBASE*, the RSNA Index of Imaging Literature, *MEDLINE/ PubMed (Index Medicus),* MEDLINE/MEDLARS, SciSearch, Research Alert, and Neuroscience Citation Index.

Printed in the United States of America.

GOAL STATEMENT

The goal of *Neuroimaging Clinics of North America* is to keep practicing radiologists and radiology residents up to date with current clinical practice in radiology by providing timely articles reviewing the state of the art in patient care.

ACCREDITATION

The *Neuroimaging Clinics of North America* is planned and implemented in accordance with the Essential Areas and Policies of the Accreditation Council for Continuing Medical Education (ACCME) through the joint sponsorship of the University of Virginia School of Medicine and Elsevier. The University of Virginia School of Medicine is accredited by the ACCME to provide continuing medical education for physicians.

The University of Virginia School of Medicine designates this educational activity for a maximum of 60 *AMA PRA Category 1 Credits*™. Physicians should only claim credit commensurate with the extent of their participation in the activity.

The American Medical Association has determined that physicians not licensed in the US who participate in this CME activity are eligible for *AMA PRA Category 1 Credits*™.

Credit can be earned by reading the text material, taking the CME examination online at http://www.theclinics.com/home/cme, and completing the evaluation. After taking the test, you will be required to review any and all incorrect answers. Following completion of the test and evaluation, your credit will be awarded and you may print your certificate.

FACULTY DISCLOSURE/CONFLICT OF INTEREST

The University of Virginia School of Medicine, as an ACCME accredited provider, endorses and strives to comply with the Accreditation Council for Continuing Medical Education (ACCME) Standards of Commercial Support, Commonwealth of Virginia statutes, University of Virginia policies and procedures, and associated federal and private regulations and guidelines on the need for disclosure and monitoring of proprietary and financial interests that may affect the scientific integrity and balance of content delivered in continuing medical education activities under our auspices.

The University of Virginia School of Medicine requires that all CME activities accredited through this institution be developed independently and be scientifically rigorous, balanced and objective in the presentation/discussion of its content, theories and practices.

All authors/editors participating in an accredited CME activity are expected to disclose to the readers relevant financial relationships with commercial entities occurring within the past 12 months (such as grants or research support, employee, consultant, stock holder, member of speakers bureau, etc.). The University of Virginia School of Medicine will employ appropriate mechanisms to resolve potential conflicts of interest to maintain the standards of fair and balanced education to the reader. Questions about specific strategies can be directed to the Office of Continuing Medical Education, University of Virginia School of Medicine, Charlottesville, Virginia.

The authors/editors listed below have identified no professional/financial affiliations for themselves or their spouse/partner:

Barton F. Branstetter, IV, MD; Ara A. Chalian, MD; Gary L. Clayman, DMD, MD, FACS; Mary Elizabeth Cunnane, MD; Saeed Fakhran, MD; Wei-Shen Griggs, MD, PhD; Amy Hessel, MD; Mohannad Ibrahim, MD; Aya Kamaya, MD; Summer L. Kaplan, MS; Jill E. Langer, MD; Laurie A. Loevner, MD (Guest Editor); Gul Moonis, MD; Jason G. Newman, MD, FACS; Daniel A. Pryma, MD; Lisa Richman (Acquiring Editor); Ashok R. Shaha, MD, FACS; Randal S. Weber, MD, FASC; and Richard O. Wein, MD, FACS.

The authors listed below have identified the following professional/financial affiliations for themselves or their spouse/partner:

Terry S. Desser, MD owns stock in Sonosite.
Chaitanya Divgi, MD is a consultant for Wilex, serves on the Speaker's bureau for GSK, and serves on the Advisory Committee for IBA.
Susan J. Mandel, MD, MPH is a speaker for Abbott Pharmaceuticals and Genzyme Corporation.
Suresh K. Mukherji, MD (Consulting Editor) is a consultant for Bracco, Bayer, Philips, and Xoran Technologies.
Hemant Parmar, MD is employed by Bayer Healthcare.

Disclosure of Discussion of non-FDA approved uses for pharmaceutical products and/or medical devices:
The University of Virginia School of Medicine, as an ACCME provider, requires that all authors/editors identify and disclose any "off label" uses for pharmaceutical products and/or for medical devices. The University of Virginia School of Medicine recommends that each reader fully review all the available data on new products or procedures prior to instituting them with patients.

TO ENROLL

To enroll in the Neuroimaging Clinics of North America Continuing Medical Education program, call customer service at 1-800-654-2452 or sign up online at **http://www.theclinics.com/home/cme**. The CME program is available to subscribers for an additional annual fee of USD 175.

Clinics in Neuroimaging

FORTHCOMING ISSUE

November 2008

Multiple Sclerosis, Volume I
Massimo Filippi, MD, *Guest Editor*

RECENT ISSUES

May 2008

Cranial Nerves
Jan Casselman, MD, PhD, *Guest Editor*

February 2008

Viruses and Prion in the CNS
E. Turgut Tali, MD, *Guest Editor*

RELATED INTEREST

Endocrinology and Metabolism Clinics of North America September 2007
Thyroid Function and Disease
Kenneth Burman, MD, *Guest Editor*
www.endo.theclinics.com

THE CLINICS ARE NOW AVAILABLE ONLINE!

Access your subscription at:
www.theclinics.com

Contributors

CONSULTING EDITOR

SURESH K. MUKHERJI, MD
Professor and Chief of Neuroradiology;
Professor of Radiology, Otolaryngology Head
Neck Surgery and Radiation Oncology,
Department of Radiology, University of
Michigan Health System, Ann Arbor, Michigan

GUEST EDITOR

LAURIE A. LOEVNER, MD
Professor of Radiology, Otorhinolaryngology:
Head and Neck Surgery and Neurosurgery,
University of Pennsylvania School of Medicine;
Department of Radiology, Neuroradiology
Division, Hospital of the University of
Pennsylvania Medical Center, Philadelphia,
Pennsylvania

AUTHORS

BARTON F. BRANSTETTER, IV, MD
Director of Head and Neck Imaging,
Department of Radiology; Department of
Otolaryngology, University of Pittsburgh,
Pittsburgh, Pennsylvania

ARA A. CHALIAN, MD
Associate Professor, Department of
Otorhinolaryngology: Head and Neck Surgery,
University of Pennsylvania Medical Center,
Philadelphia, Pennsylvania

GARY L. CLAYMAN, DMD, MD, FACS
Professor, The Department of Head and Neck
Surgery, The University of Texas M. D.
Anderson Cancer Center, Houston, Texas

MARY ELIZABETH CUNNANE, MD
Department of Radiology, Massachusetts Eye
and Ear Infirmary, Boston, Massachusetts

TERRY S. DESSER, MD
Associate Professor, Department of Radiology,
Stanford University School of Medicine,
Stanford, California

CHAITANYA DIVGI, MD
Professor of Radiology; Professor of Radiation
Oncology, Wistar Institute; Abramson Cancer
Center, University of Pennsylvania; Nuclear
Medicine and Clinical Molecular Imaging,
Hospital of the University of Pennsylvania,
Philadelphia, Pennsylvania

SAEED FAKHRAN, MD
Department of Radiology, University of
Pittsburgh, Pittsburgh, Pennsylvania

WEI-SHEN GRIGGS, MD, PhD
Staff Radiologist, Fairfax Radiological
Consultants, Fairfax, Virginia

Contributors

AMY HESSEL, MD
Assistant Professor, The Department of Head and Neck Surgery, The University of Texas, M.D. Anderson Cancer Center, Houston, Texas

MOHANNAD IBRAHIM, MD
Division of Neuroradiology, Department of Radiology, University of Michigan Health System, University of Michigan, Ann Arbor, Michigan

AYA KAMAYA, MD
Assistant Professor, Department of Radiology, Stanford University School of Medicine, Stanford, California

SUMMER L. KAPLAN, MS
University of Pennsylvania School of Medicine, Philadelphia, Pennsylvania

JILL E. LANGER, MD
Associate Professor of Radiology, Department of Radiology, University of Pennsylvania School of Medicine, Hospital of the University of Pennsylvania, Philadelphia, Pennsylvania

LAURIE A. LOEVNER, MD
Professor of Radiology, Otorhinolaryngology: Head and Neck Surgery and Neurosurgery, University of Pennsylvania School of Medicine; Department of Radiology, Neuroradiology Division, Hospital of the University of Pennsylvania Medical Center, Philadelphia, Pennsylvania

SUSAN J. MANDEL, MD, MPH
Associate Professor of Medicine, Division of Endocrinology, Diabetes, and Metabolism, Department of Medicine, University of Pennsylvania School of Medicine, Philadelphia, Pennsylvania

GUL MOONIS, MD
Department of Radiology, Beth Israel Deaconess Medical Center, Boston, Massachusetts

JASON G. NEWMAN, MD, FACS
Assistant Professor, Department of Otorhinolaryngology, Head and Neck Surgery, Center for Cranial Base Surgery, University of Pennsylvania, Pennsylvania Hospital, Philadelphia, Pennsylvania

HEMANT PARMAR, MD
Division of Neuroradiology, Department of Radiology, University of Michigan Health System, University of Michigan, Ann Arbor, Michigan

DANIEL A. PRYMA, MD
Division of Nuclear Medicine and Clinical Molecular Imaging, Department of Radiology, University of Pennsylvania, Philadelphia, Pennsylvania

ASHOK R. SHAHA, MD, FACS
Professor of Surgery, Cornell University Medical College; Memorial Sloan-Kettering Cancer Center, New York, New York

RANDAL S. WEBER, MD, FACS
Professor and Chairman, Department of Head and Neck Surgery, University of Texas M.D. Anderson Cancer Center, Houston, Texas

RICHARD O. WEIN, MD, FACS
Assistant Professor, Department of Otolaryngology–Head and Neck Surgery, Tufts Medical Center, Boston, Massachusetts

Contents

Foreword xi

Suresh K. Mukherji

Preface xiii

Laurie A. Loevner

Cross-Sectional Imaging of the Thyroid Gland 445

Laurie A. Loevner, Summer L. Kaplan, Mary Elizabeth Cunnane, and Gul Moonis

> Directed imaging is useful in assessing the thyroid gland. Nuclear scintigraphy reveals functional information about the thyroid gland, while cross-sectional imaging, including ultrasound, CT, and MR imaging provide important adjunctive anatomic information about the thyroid as well as about related structures in the neck, including the presence or absence of cervical and mediastinal lymphadenopathy, or extension of thyroid disease into adjacent soft tissues or the mediastinum. This article reviews the anatomy and physiology of the thyroid gland and addresses issues related to diseases affecting the thyroid gland, with an emphasis on neoplasms and the role of cross-sectional MR and CT imaging in the assessment of thyroid neoplasia.

Ultrasound of Thyroid Nodules 463

Terry S. Desser and Aya Kamaya

> Thyroid nodules can be detected in 4% to 8% of the adult population by palpation, but in 40% to 50% of the population by ultrasound. The overwhelming majority of these represent benign hyperplastic nodules or adenomas. Approximately 5% of nodules are malignant, with papillary carcinoma representing approximately 75% to 80% of primary thyroid malignancies. Although many sonographic features have been studied as a means of distinguishing benign from malignant nodules, ultrasound-guided fine-needle aspiration with cytologic evaluation remains a mainstay in the management of palpable and incidentally detected nodules. This article reviews the current techniques for sonographic evaluation of the thyroid and the imaging features of the various types of thyroid nodules.

Sonographic Imaging of Cervical Lymph Nodes in Patients with Thyroid Cancer 479

Jill E. Langer and Susan J. Mandel

> Sonography plays an important role in the evaluation of patients who have thyroid carcinoma by identifying metastatic disease to the regional cervical lymph nodes. The sonographic appearance of lymph node metastases may vary from subtle alterations in echogenicity or vascular patterns to more obvious findings of calcifications and cystic changes within an affected node. Identification of metastatic disease to

lateral cervical lymph nodes by sonography may affect the extent of surgical resection at the time of diagnosis. In patients who have had thyroidectomy for cancer, sonographic evaluation has proved to be the most sensitive imaging technique to detect thyroid cancer recurrence in the neck.

Surgical Approaches in Thyroid Cancer: What the Radiologist Needs to Know 491

Jason G. Newman, Ara A. Chalian, and Ashok R. Shaha

This article discusses the broad topic of thyroid cancer, with a focus on giving the reader an understanding of the basis for surgical decision making. The reader will gain an understanding of the embryology, anatomy, and various cancer pathologies than can affect the thyroid gland. The reader will also be exposed to clinical correlations that greatly assist in management of these cancers. Planning and rationale for various surgical procedures are also discussed.

Radioiodine Imaging and Treatment in Thyroid Disorders 505

Wei-Shen Griggs and Chaitanya Divgi

The thyroid produces thyroid hormones that regulate metabolism and are essential to proper development and differentiation of the cells in the body. Iodine is an essential element in thyroid hormone synthesis. The thyroid has the ability to concentrate and incorporate iodine into thyroid hormone. Incorporation of iodine is essential to the formation of thyroid hormone. Thyroid disorders may be imaged and treated with radioiodine. Iodine uptake by thyroid follicular cells lends itself to imaging of functional characteristics of the gland. Gamma camera and, increasingly, PET imaging of thyroid disorders permit delineation of thyroid functional status. Iodine uptake also permits treatment, using I-131, of hyperthyroid disease and cancer, for which I-131 is the primary treatment.

Surgical Management of Recurrent Thyroid Cancer 517

Amy Hessel, Ara A. Chalian, and Gary L. Clayman

While well-differentiated thyroid cancer is generally thought to be a treatable cancer with excellent outcomes, some patients suffer from recurrent disease. Risk factors for recurrent disease include primary disease greater than 4 cm, incomplete resection, multiple positive lymph nodes in the central compartment, and lateral neck disease with multiple positive lymph nodes in multiple levels or pathologic extracapsular extension. These factors can help stratify the thyroid cancer population in to low-, medium-, and high-risk patients. Low-risk patients can generally be followed with thyroglogulin levels and routine ultrasounds to the head and neck. High-risk patients are best monitored with stimulated thyroglobulin, ultrasound of the head and neck, and low-dose iodine 131 uptake scans at the 6- to 12-month mark. The treatment of locoregional recurrent thyroid cancer is surgical resection with the overall goal of complete tumor removal while maintaining function and decreasing risks. The use of adjuvant therapy is dependent on the presence / absence of high risk pathologic features.

Extrathyroidal Manifestations of Thyroid Disease: Thyroid Ophthalmopathy 527

Hemant Parmar and Mohannad Ibrahim

Thyroid ophthalmopathy is a common autoimmune, inflammatory disease involving the orbit. Diagnosis is based on the clinical presentation and findings. Imaging, mainly CT and MR imaging, are helpful to reveal the extent of disease and degree of muscle enlargement and to evaluate for complications, such as optic nerve compression. This article reviews the basic pathology and pathophysiology of the disease and describes the extensive imaging findings on CT and MR imaging. The differential diagnosis of thyroid ophthalmopathy is reviewed.

Parathyroid Imaging 537

Saeed Fakhran, Barton F. Branstetter, and Daniel A. Pryma

The most common indication for parathyroid imaging is hyperparathyroidism, which is caused by a solitary parathyroid adenoma in most patients. The primary function of parathyroid imaging is localization of the abnormal parathyroid gland, enabling the surgeon to pursue a minimally invasive resection. Ultrasound and ^{99m}Tc sestamibi scintigraphy are the mainstays for the preoperative localization of culprit lesions. The emerging modality of SPECT-CT can improve the sensitivity of ^{99m}Tc sestamibi scintigraphy and its use is encouraged when available. CT and MR imaging are useful as adjuncts, particularly as anatomic correlates to suspected ectopic glands on ^{99m}Tc sestamibi scintigraphy that are inaccessible to ultrasound. In cases of suspected parathyroid carcinoma, preoperative CT or MR imaging is recommended for surgical planning.

Parathyroid Surgery: What the Radiologists Need to Know 551

Richard O. Wein and Randal S. Weber

Hyperparathyroidism represents by a varied spectrum of presentations, from those individuals who have overt symptoms directly attributable to hypercalcemia to those who are asymptomatic at diagnosis. Indications for surgical intervention in the asymptomatic population have changed as the long-term experience with these patients has grown. Use of additional imaging techniques to aid localization and a detailed understanding of the anatomy can be critical to a successful operative outcome. This article discusses the pertinent issues that surround the current surgical management of parathyroid disease with a focus on epidemiology, surgical anatomy, and operative strategies.

Index 559

Foreword

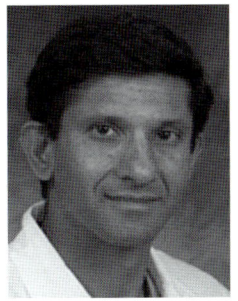

Suresh K. Mukherji, MD
Consulting Editor

In the preface, Laurie says that she "was delighted when approached to edit this issue on the thyroid and parathyroid glands for *Neuroimaging Clinics of North America*." Well, if she was "delighted," then I was super-duper delighted when she accepted! Laurie Loevner, MD, is Professor of Radiology and Head and Neck Radiology at the University of Pennsylvania. Dr. Loevner is an authority in head and neck imaging and is recognized as one of the premier head and neck radiologists in the world. She is a tireless worker who is always overcommitted yet always manages to deliver. She is also the living example of the adage that "if you really want something done, give it to the busiest person!" Besides being a professional colleague for many years, I am very happy to have her as a friend as well.

The thyroid gland is located in the neck, however, neuroradiologists and head and neck radiologists tend not to focus on disorders involving the gland. Instead, the thyroid gland is often considered a no-person's land because numerous modalities and referring physicians are involved in the diagnosis, management, and treatment of glandular disorders. The initial diagnosis of a thyroid mass is often an incidental finding identified on a routine physical exam. A thyroid nodule may also be incidentally detected on an imaging study (CT, MR, or PET-CT) performed for unrelated reasons. As a result, subsequent imaging studies often vary depending on how the thyroid mass was initially diagnosed, the histology, and other associated clinical findings. The treatment and management may also involve numerous medical specialties, including general surgeons, endocrine surgeons, head and neck surgeons, endocrinologists, ultrasonographers, neuroradiologists, and nuclear medicine physicians. Because of these complexities, it is often difficult for radiologists to understand the nuances for thyroid disorders.

This edition is a concise, yet comprehensive, text that covers the diagnosis, management, and treatment of a variety of thyroid and parathyroid diseases. Dr. Loevenr has done an outstanding job putting together this issue. Her invited authors include ultrasonographers, neuroradiologists, nuclear medicine physicians, endocrinologists, and ENT surgeons who are recognized experts in thyroid and parathyroid imaging. I wish to personally thank Dr. Loevner and all of her coauthors for creating an outstanding and comprehensive state-of-the-art issue that will serve as a excellent reference on the thyroid and parathyroid gland for many years to come.

Suresh K. Mukherji, MD
Neuroradiology Radiology, Otolaryngology Head
Neck Surgery and Radiation Oncology
Department of Radiology
University of Michigan Health System
UH B2A209B
1500 East Medical Center Drive
Ann Arbor, MI 48109-5030, USA

E-mail address:
mukherji@med.umich.edu (S.K. Mukherji)

Preface

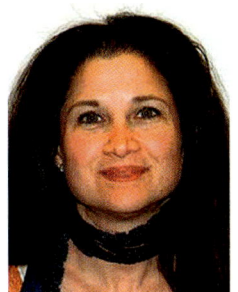

Laurie A. Loevner, MD
Guest Editor

I was delighted when approached to edit this issue on the thyroid and parathyroid glands for *Neuroimaging Clinics of North America*. I have entitled this issue "Thyroid and Parathyroid Glands: Imaging, Treatment and Beyond," which accurately reflects its contents, thanks to the significant contributions of so many talented authors and coauthors who are highly recognized for their expertise in these areas. I have tried to focus this issue on the evaluation of thyroid nodules and thyroid nodules that are cancer, followed by the evaluation of the parathyroid glands with an emphasis on localizing parathyroid adenomas and surgical approaches for resection. The nationally recognized authors in this issue are from all over the continent, east to west, and reflect the outstanding work from many wonderful academic institutions. Importantly, this issue is multidisciplinary, reflecting the essential teamwork necessary to adequately diagnose and treat pathology of the thyroid and parathyroid glands. There are contributions from ultrasonographers, neuroradiologists, physicians who image and treat thyroid cancer using radionuclides, endocrinologists, and ENT surgeons.

In our introductory article, my coauthors and I review the essential embryology, anatomy, and physiology of the thyroid gland. This is followed by a discussion on the radiologist's imaging arsenal in assessing thyroid disease, thyroid nodules, and thyroid cancer. The introductory article finishes with a focused discussion on when to perform cross-sectional imaging (CT, MRI, and PET) in newly diagnosed and recurrent thyroid cancer. Ultrasound of thyroid nodules, indications for ultrasound-guided fine-needle aspiration, and how to work up cancerous nodules are covered with great attention to detail by Drs. Desser and Kamaya. In the third article, sonographic imaging of cervical lymph nodes in patients with thyroid cancer is covered with great expertise by the combined efforts of Drs. Langer and Mandel, an ultrasonographer and an endocrinologist, respectively.

Next, this issue covers the surgical approaches for newly diagnosed and recurrent thyroid cancer, which are discussed with an emphasis on providing radiologists with the information they need to effectively assist their clinical and surgical colleagues in the appropriate management of patients with thyroid cancer. Dr. Jason Newman, a head and neck cancer surgeon, and his coauthors Drs. Chalian and Shaha, discuss thyroid cancer with a focus on understanding the basis for surgical decision making. The spectrum of cancer pathologies that affect the thyroid gland, clinical correlations that assist in management of these cancers, and the planning rationale for various surgical procedures are discussed. Dr. Amy Hessel and coauthors Drs. Chalian and Clayman specifically address the surgical management of recurrent thyroid cancer. In their article, these ENT surgeons also discuss the epidemiology and risk factors for persistent and recurrent thyroid cancer and provide some possible approaches for localizing recurrences. The last article in this section focuses on the imaging and treatment of thyroid disorders using radionuclides, with an emphasis on cancer. Drs. Griggs and Divgi review instrumentation and techniques, patient preparation, as well as nuclear imaging and radioablation in thyroid diseases.

The next article by Dr. Parmar covers the extra–thyroidal manifestations of thyroid disease with an emphasis on thyroid ophthalmopathy. In this article, the basic pathology and pathophysiology of this disease and its diagnosis, including applications of CT and MR imaging, are reviewed. Also discussed are treatment options.

The last two articles of this issue focus on the parathyroid glands. Dr. Saeed Fakhran and coauthors discuss the pathophysiology of hyperparathyroidism, the evolving role of imaging in parathyroid localization, and the potential pitfalls of the radiologist's arsenal. To close out this issue, ENT surgeons Drs. Richard Wein and Randal Weber focus on understanding the basis for surgical decision making in parathyroid surgery.

Throughout this issue, radiologists and a spectrum of clinicians work together to provide a rational approach for the evaluation and multidisciplinary care of patients with diseases affecting the thyroid and parathyroid glands. I hope readers will find the following pages as informative and educational as I believe them to be. Most importantly, I hope you enjoy reading them as much as I did.

Laurie A. Loevner, MD
Department of Radiology
Neuroradiology Division
Hospital of the University of Pennsylvania
Medical Center
3400 Spruce Street
2nd Floor Dulles, Suite 219
Philadelphia, PA 19104

E-mail address:
laurie.loevner@uphs.upenn.edu (L.A. Loevner)

Cross-Sectional Imaging of the Thyroid Gland

Laurie A. Loevner, MD[a,b,*], Summer L. Kaplan, MS[c],
Mary Elizabeth Cunnane, MD[d], Gul Moonis, MD[e]

KEYWORDS

- Thyroid gland • Ultrasound • CT • MRI • Radioablation
- Thyroid surgery • Parathyroid localization
- Parathyroid surgery • Sestamibi • Radionuclides

The thyroid gland plays an important role in the regulation of many metabolic functions, including cardiac rate, lipid metabolism, skeletal growth, and heat production. As a result, the evaluation of patients with hypo- or hyperthyroidism requires an understanding of the hormonal functions that the thyroid gland performs. Thyroid nodules are detected by physical examination in up to 7% of the United States population. While the majority of nodules are benign, 7% to 10% represent thyroid carcinomas.

Directed imaging is useful in assessing the thyroid gland. Nuclear scintigraphy reveals functional information about the thyroid gland, while cross-sectional imaging, including ultrasound, CT, and MR imaging, provide important adjunctive anatomic information about the thyroid as well as about related structures in the neck, including the presence or absence of cervical and mediastinal lymphadenopathy, or extension of thyroid disease into adjacent soft tissues or the mediastinum.

This article reviews the anatomy and physiology of the thyroid gland and addresses Issues related to diseases affecting the thyroid gland, with an emphasis on neoplasms and the role of cross-sectional MR and CT imaging in the assessment of thyroid neoplasia.

DEVELOPMENT AND ANATOMY OF THE THYROID GLAND

The thyroid gland develops in the first trimester of pregnancy, beginning around the fifth week of gestation, and is completed by the 10th gestational week. It develops from median and paired lateral anlages. The median anlage arises in the midline oropharynx at the fourth to fifth gestational week and gives rise to follicular thyroid tissue, which will secrete hormones.[1] The lateral anlages are believed to arise from the ultimobranchial bodies, which are derived from the fourth and fifth branchial pharyngeal pouches at around the fifth week of gestation. They give rise to the parafollicular C-cells, which will secrete calcitonin and are thought to derive from the neural crest.[1] By the 10th week in utero, the right and left lateral anlages fuse with the median anlage, resulting in the bilobed thyroid gland.[1,2]

During fetal development, the thyroid gland descends from its place of origin, the foramen cecum at the base of the tongue, to its final adult destination in the lower neck. The thyroid is attached to the tongue base by the thyroglossal duct, which is lined by squamous epithelium. During the caudal descent of the gland, this duct elongates and

---

[a] Otorhinolaryngology: Head and Neck Surgery and Neurosurgery, University of Pennsylvania School of Medicine, 3400 Spruce Street, Philadelphia, PA 19104, USA
[b] Department of Radiology, Neuroradiology Division, Hospital of the University of Pennsylvania Medical Center, 3400 Spruce Street, Philadelphia, PA 19104, USA
[c] University of Pennsylvania School of Medicine, 3400 Spruce Street, Philadelphia, PA 19104, USA
[d] Department of Radiology, Massachusetts Eye and Ear Infirmary, 243 Charles Street, Boston, MA 02114, USA
[e] Department of Radiology, Beth Israel Deaconess Medical Center, 330 Brookline Avenue, Boston, MA 02215, USA
* Corresponding author. Department of Radiology, Neuroradiology Division, Hospital of the University of Pennsylvania, 3400 Spruce Street, 2nd floor Dulles, Suite 219, Philadelphia, PA 19104.
E-mail address: laurie.loevner@uphs.upenn.edu (L.A. Loevner).

subsequently degenerates. Abnormal development or aberrant caudal descent of the thyroid gland results in a spectrum of anomalies. Arrest of descent can occur anywhere from the tongue down to the lower neck. Failure of descent of the median thyroid anlage, or complete failure of descent of the thyroid, results in a lingual thyroid at the base of the tongue, the most common type of functioning ectopic thyroid tissue. In these cases, up to 75% of patients may have no functioning thyroid tissue in the neck.[3–5] Overdescent of the thyroid may result in ectopic thyroid in the lower neck, in the mediastinum, or within mediastinal structures. On rare occasions, thyroid tissue may be found in the trachea,[6] in the heart, or within ovarian teratomas (struma ovarii).[7,8] Any pathology that may arise within normally located thyroid may also arise in ectopic tissue. Other developmental anomalies of the thyroid gland include agenesis or hemiagenesis (most often the left lobe) with normal formation of the contralateral lobe and isthmus.[9–12]

The thyroid gland is shield-shaped and consists of right and left lobes adjoined by the isthmus, though occasionally the isthmus may be absent. The thyroid isthmus is anterior to the trachea (usually overlying the first through third tracheal rings). Infrequently, it may reside anterior to the cricoid cartilage. The thyroid is anterior to the prevertebral and paraspinal musculature, and deep to the sternothyroid and sternohyoid muscles. Usually, the thyroid gland terminates above the clavicles. However, substernal extension into the superior mediastinum may occur. An accessory lobe, the pyramidal lobe, may be present in 50% to 70% of people and usually arises from the isthmus and extends superiorly along the course of the distal thyroglossal duct.[13] It may be attached to the hyoid bone. Uncommonly, the pyramidal lobe may arise from the medial right or left thyroid lobe. A pyramidal lobe is most commonly recognized in patients with Graves' disease.

The visceral fascia, part of the middle layer of the deep cervical fascia, attaches the thyroid gland to the larynx and trachea. As a result, the gland or abnormalities related to it will move with the larynx during swallowing. The thyroid gland is encapsulated, and septae from the capsule extend into the substance of the gland.

The thyroid gland has a rich vascular supply with paired (right and left) superior and inferior thyroidal arteries. The superior thyroidal arteries are the first branches from the respective external carotid arteries, and travel inferiorly to the thyroid gland. The thyrocervical trunks originate from the subclavian arteries, and each gives rise to an inferior thyroidal artery. The thyroidea ima is an inconstant artery that arises directly from the aortic arch and helps supply the inferior thyroid gland. Superior and middle thyroidal veins drain into the internal jugular veins, and inferior veins drain into the innominate vein. The vagus nerve and the cervical sympathetic plexus innervate the thyroid gland. Sympathetic fibers descend from the sympathetic trunk, while parasympathetic fibers are along the course of the vagus nerve. This autonomic innervation is felt to strongly influence perfusion to the thyroid gland.

ENDOCRINOLOGY OF THE THYROID GLAND

The thyroid gland contains multiple lobules, each composed of multiple follicles. In these follicles, thyroglobulin is stored within colloid, and the follicular cells secrete hormones. Parafollicular (C) cells are dispersed throughout the stroma of the gland and secrete thyrocalcitonin. The primary function of the thyroid gland is the synthesis of hormones that regulate numerous metabolic functions. Two hormones, triiodothyronine (T3) and thyroxine (T4) are synthesized within the thyroid gland and released in response to a feedback mechanism with the pituitary-hypothalamic axis.

The synthesis of hormones within the thyroid is a regulated, systematic process. The first step involves trapping of iodide from the circulating plasma via active transport into the thyroid gland, where it is concentrated within follicular cells, and oxidized by thyroid peroxidase into its chemically active form. Subsequently, organification occurs. In this process, tyrosine residues on thyroglobulin molecules are iodinated to form monoiodotyrosine (MIT) and diiodotyrosine (DIT). The coupling of MIT and DIT forms T3, and the coupling of two molecules of DIT forms T4. T3 and T4 are released from thyroglobulin and secreted into the circulation in free and bound forms.[14] Simultaneously, deiodination of free MIT and DIT occurs for iodide salvage and recycling within the thyroid gland. Aberrant organification usually results from enzymatic defects that interfere with the oxidation of iodide or the iodination of tyrosine. Iodide trapping may fail, but this is rare.

In the circulation, carrier proteins transport thyroid hormones. T4-binding globulin carries approximately 70% of T3 and T4, T4-binding preglobulin carries about 5% of T3 and 25% of T4, and albumin carries the remaining hormones. The active form of T3 and T4 is the free unbound form, representing only 0.3% of T3 and 0.03% of T4. T4 is synthesized entirely within the thyroid, while 80% of T3 is synthesized by peripheral conversion of T4 in the liver and muscle.

Several medications may temporarily interfere with the intrathyroidal transport or organification of iodide, including iodinated contrast materials frequently used in CT studies; oral cholecystographic agents; T4; liothyronine; antithyroid medications, such as propylthiouracil and methimazole; and amiodarone. These will alter radioactive iodine uptake in nuclear scintigraphy studies.

CLINICAL MANIFESTATIONS OF THYROID DISEASE

Thyrotoxicosis is a clinical syndrome that develops when circulating levels of T4 and T3 are increased (thyrotropin is usually suppressed). Hyperthyroidism refers to sustained thyroid hyperfunction with increased thyroid hormone synthesis and release. Symptoms of thyrotoxicosis include warmth and flushing due to peripheral vasodilatation, heat loss, weight loss, myopathy, and increased appetite. Patients, especially children, may be hyperactive. Cardiac manifestations are more common in older patients and include tachycardia, palpitations, arrhythmias, and cardiomegaly.

Thyrotoxicosis associated with hyperthyroidism is most frequently seen with Graves' disease, but may be seen with toxic multinodular goiter, and rarely a hyperfunctioning thyrotropin-secreting pituitary adenoma or thyroid neoplasm. Toxic multinodular goiter associated with hyperthyroidism (Plummer's disease) commonly develops after 50 years of age and is related to a hyperfunctioning thyroid nodule.[15] Thyrotoxicosis not associated with hyperthyroidism (low radioactive-iodine uptake) may be related to inflammatory thyroid disease or ectopic thyroid tissue (ovarian strumii), or it may be factitious (exogenous hormone use) (**Box 1**).

Thyroid ophthalmopathy, more common in women, is characterized by enlargement of the bellies of the extraocular muscles with sparing of the tendinous insertions, and is most commonly seen in Graves' disease. The most common patterns of extraocular involvement are enlargement of all of the muscles, or of the inferior and medial muscle complexes.[16] Isolated involvement of the lateral rectus muscle is rare and when present should raise suspicion for a different disease process, such as myositis or pseudotumor. Clinical signs and symptoms of thyroid ophthalmopathy include unilateral or bilateral proptosis due to increased orbital fat and an increase in the volume of the extraocular muscles related to edema and lymphocytic infiltrates, lid retraction that may result in corneal exposure, and decreased eye motion.[16] Extraocular muscle enlargement may cause compression of the optic nerve at the orbital apex resulting in visual loss, which may require surgical decompression if refractory to medical therapy. Late in disease, contractures, fatty infiltration, and fibrosis of the extraocular muscles may lead to abnormal eye movements.

Hypothyroidism refers to decreased thyroid hormone synthesis with low T3 and T4 levels (serum thyrotropin is usually high). Primary hypothyroidism may be due to structural or functional abnormalities of the thyroid gland. In adults, this most often results from processes that destroy thyroid tissue, such as autoimmune disease or iodine 131 (I-131) treatment. In children, it may be related to enzyme deficiencies, defects in organification, or congenital anomalies, such as lingual thyroid or thyroid agenesis.[10] Central hypothyroidism results from decreased thyroid stimulation by thyrotropin related to pituitary disease (secondary hypothyroidism) or hypothalamic thyrotropin-releasing hormone deficiency (tertiary hypothyroidism). Serum thyrotropin levels are normal in the presence of low serum T3 and T4 concentrations. Hypothyroidism occurring in the prenatal period or during infancy results in cretinism if not readily identified and treated. Hypothyroidism in older children and adults (myxedema) has variable clinical manifestations ranging from fatigue to coma, depending upon the degree and duration of hypothyroidism.

Secondary manifestations of thyroid disease are frequently responsible for clinical presentation. Marked enlargement of the thyroid gland most common in multinodular goiter, but also seen in neoplastic and inflammatory processes, may compress the adjacent esophagus, causing

---

Box 1
Evaluation of the hyperthyroid patient

Elevated thyroid function tests and normal 24-hour radioactive iodine uptake (10%–30%)

Plummer's disease

Graves' disease

Elevated thyroid function tests and low 24-hour radioactive iodine uptake (<10%)

Thyroiditis

De Quervain's

Subacute lymphocytic

Struma ovarii

Factitious

Elevated thyroid function tests and high 24-hour radioactive iodine uptake (>30%)

Graves' disease

Plummer's disease

dysphasia, and trachea, causing respiratory distress. The recurrent laryngeal nerve travels in the tracheoesophageal groove, and thyroid lesions that affect this area may present with vocal cord paralysis. Cervical lymphadenopathy in the presence of a thyroid mass, or extension of a thyroid mass outside the capsule into adjacent structures, such as the trachea, is usually indicative of thyroid neoplasia.

IMAGING THE THYROID GLAND: THE RADIOLOGIST'S ARSENAL
Nuclear Scintigraphy

Nuclear scintigraphy provides excellent functional information about the thyroid gland because the radionuclides used to image the gland do so by using some step of hormone synthesis in the thyroid gland. The primary role of scintigraphy is in the evaluation of patients with tests that show abnormal thyroid function, especially hyperthyroidism. Scintigraphy determines if the cause of hyperthyroidism is a diffuse process, such as Graves' disease, or an autonomously functioning nodule. Scintigraphy of a focal thyroid mass in a euthyroid patient may determine whether a lesion is functioning (very low incidence of malignancy) or nonfunctioning "cold," a feature carrying a reported risk of malignancy ranging from 8% to 25%.[9,17] However, 95% of thyroid nodules are cold and, hence, nuclear scintigraphy plays a minor role in the workup of dominant thyroid nodules.

Morphologic detail of the thyroid gland is obtained using technetium (Tc-99m) pertechnetate or iodine 123 (I-123). Tc-99m is trapped by the thyroid allowing an estimate of thyroid activity, whereas I-123 is also organified providing a true assessment of diffuse or focal regions of uptake.[18] For routes of administration and doses of radionuclides see **Table 1**. Imaging is performed approximately 20 minutes following administration of Tc-99m pertechnetate, 4 to 24 hours after oral ingestion of I-123, and 24 to 72 hours following administration of I-131. The normal thyroid gland shows homogenous radionuclide uptake. The isthmus may demonstrate slightly less activity than the thyroid lobes.

I-123 is used for obtaining the 24-hour thyroid iodine uptake. Thyroid uptake reflects the percentage of the dose given to the patient that is accumulated within the gland, corrected for radioactive decay. Normal 24-hour uptake ranges from 10% to 30%. Several medications, iodine-containing topical solutions, and intravenous iodinated contrast agents used for imaging may temporarily interfere with the organification of iodide, altering radioactive iodine uptake measurements for as long as 6 weeks.[19–22] The uptake of radioactive iodine may be reduced by as much as 50% 1 week following injection of iodinated contrast for a CT scan.[19–21] In over one third of patients with underlying thyroid disease, temporary changes in thyroid function may occur following injection of iodinated contrast material.[19] Therefore, if cross-sectional imaging is felt to be necessary in a patient who will also be studied with nuclear scans using iodinated radionuclides, MR imaging can be obtained. If the patient has a contraindication for MR imaging, then CT should be performed without intravenous contrast administration and, if contrast is desired, the CT should be performed following evaluation with nuclear scintigraphy.

Iodinated radionuclides may be used both in the imaging evaluation and treatment of patients with

Table 1
Radionuclides used in thyroid gland imaging and treatment of thyroid cancer

Radionuclide	Administration	Dose	Half-life
Tc-99m	Intravenous	74–370 MBq	6.02 h
I-123	Oral	7.4–14.8 MBq	13.6 h
I-131 (diagnostic)	Oral	1.11–3.7 MBq	8.05 d
I-131 (whole body)[a]	Oral	74–185 MBq	—
I-123 (whole body)[a]	Oral	37–92.5 MBq	—
I-131 (treatment)[b]	Oral	3700 MBq	—
I-131 (treatment)[c]	Oral	3700–7400 MBq	—

[a] Diagnostic whole-body scan following thyroidectomy to evaluate for residual thyroid tissue, or to detect metastases; to detect ectopic thyroid tissue, such as struma ovarii, in hyperthyroid patients with no demonstrable iodine uptake in the thyroid.
[b] Cancer treatment following thyroidectomy to ablate residual thyroid tissue (may require hospital admission, depending on dose).
[c] Cancer treatment to ablate thyroid metastases (may require hospital admission, depending on dose).

thyroid cancers that concentrate iodine. They are particularly useful in the follow-up of patients after thyroidectomy to evaluate for residual thyroid tissue in the operative bed, as well as to assess for recurrent or distant metastatic disease (see thyroid malignancies).

Fluorine-18-labeled fluorodeoxyglucose (FDG) positron emission tomography (PET) is playing an increasing role in the evaluation of select patients treated for thyroid cancer. It may be particularly useful in metastatic thyroid tumors that do not concentrate radioiodine.[23,24] It is increasingly used in the workup of rising serum thyroglobulin levels in patients following thyroidectomy with clinically negative examinations, and is valuable in increasing physician confidence in the detection of disease as well as in the planning of management of recurrent disease.[25] Whole-body scans are obtained to identify regions of FDG uptake. Potential pitfalls include indolent or well-differentiated thyroid tumors that take-up FDG poorly, and FDG uptake that may not be related to metastatic thyroid cancer.

Ultrasonography

Sonography is the primary imaging modality for the evaluation of thyroid disease. Compared with other imaging modalities sonography provides the highest resolution and therefore is best able to detect and characterize diffuse and focal thyroid abnormalities.[26,27] Ultrasound may also be used to guide fine needle aspiration of nodular disease within the thyroid (**Fig. 1**), or to guide aspiration of suspicious cervical lymph nodes in the setting of thyroid cancer.[28–30]

Real-time ultrasound is usually performed with a high-resolution linear array transducer ranging from 7.5 to 12 MHz.[31] The patient is placed in a supine position and the neck is mildly hyperextended. The thyroid gland is imaged in its entirety both in transverse and longitudinal planes. The carotid arteries and jugular veins are posterior and lateral to the thyroid lobes, respectively, and provide excellent anatomic markers during the examination. The examination also includes assessment of the midline neck from the sternal notch to the hyoid bone to detect lesions, such as thyroglossal duct cysts. The normal thyroid gland is uniformly hyperechoic relative to the strap muscles and homogeneous in echotexture (**Fig. 2**).[31] The superior and inferior thyroidal arteries and veins and their intrathyroidal branches are often identified.

Limitations of sonography include the skill of the operator; the inability of sonography to assess the deep structures of the neck, such as the skull base; and limited detection of retrotracheal and intrathoracic extension of an enlarged thyroid due to acoustic impedance caused by air in the trachea or adjacent bones. Ultrasound is also limited in detecting extension of thyroid malignancy into the trachea, esophagus, or other adjacent soft tissue structures of the neck.

Cross-Sectional Imaging: CT and MR Imaging

CT and MR imaging provide important adjunctive anatomic information in select clinical scenarios, especially in assessing advanced thyroid carcinomas at presentation, as well as in the evaluation of recurrent thyroid cancer following thyroidectomy. These modalities may play a critical role in the detection of lymph node metastases, especially nodal metastases in clinically occult areas that are poorly assessed by ultrasound (retropharynx and mediastinum), and are critical in evaluating extension of thyroid disease into adjacent tissues

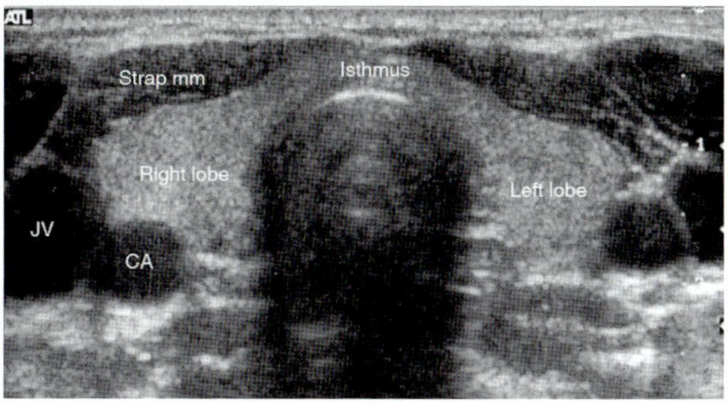

Fig. 1. Ultrasound of normal thyroid gland. The normal thyroid gland is uniformly hyperechoic relative to the strap muscles and homogeneous in background echotexture. The surface of the thyroid is smooth and demarcated from the adjacent structures by the overlying thin capsule. CA, common carotid artery; JV, jugular vein; mm, muscles.

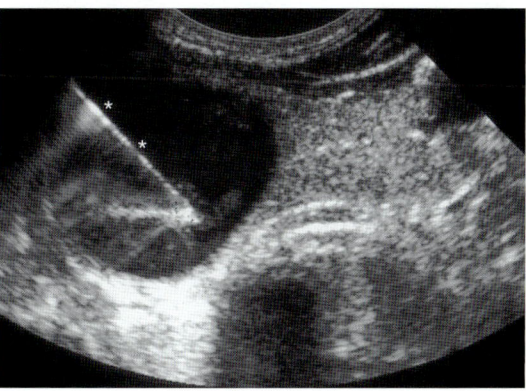

Fig. 2. Ultrasound study of a dominant thyroid nodule shows a needle (*double asterisks*) in the complex solid and cystic thyroid mass.

in the neck. Specifically, these modalities accommodate assessments of invasion of the adjacent musculature, esophagus, trachea/larynx, and jugular vein (**Fig. 3**).[26] The information provided by CT and MR imaging in these cases is invaluable in planning the surgical approach.

Because of its iodide content, the normal thyroid gland has a density of 80 to 100 Hounsfield units on CT. The intravenous injection of iodinated contrast material usually diffusely increases the density of the gland. Iodinated contrast material may provide additional information about thyroid lesions. However, because the contrast contains iodine, it will alter radioactive iodine uptake measurements for up to 6 weeks following the study. Therefore, in patients in whom nuclear scintigraphy is also going to be performed, contrast should not be administered. If both functional and cross-sectional studies are felt to be necessary, nuclear imaging can be performed before CT, or MR imaging may be used in conjunction with scintigraphy, as the contrast agent used in MR (gadolinium) does not interfere with iodide uptake or organification by the thyroid.

Imaging of the thyroid gland with MR should be multiplanar with multiple pulse sequences, including unenhanced sagittal and axial T1-weighted (T1-W) images, as well as axial fast spin-echo T2-weighted (T2-W) images with the application of fat saturation. Following the intravenous administration of gadolinium, axial T1-W images with the application of fat saturation are acquired. Because lesions may be hyperintense (bright) and fat in the neck is hyperintense on T1-W and T2-W images, fat-suppression helps to increase lesion conspicuity. On T1-W images, the normal thyroid gland shows homogeneous signal intensity slightly greater than that of the neck musculature. On T2-W images, the thyroid gland is hyperintense relative to the neck musculature. Following contrast administration, the normal gland enhances homogenously.

NODULAR DISEASES OF THE THYROID GLAND
Thyroid Goiter

Goiter refers to any enlargement of the thyroid gland. Nodular goiter is characterized by excessive growth with structural or functional transformation of one or several areas within an otherwise normal gland. In the absence of autoimmune thyroid disease, thyroiditis, thyroid dysfunction, and thyroid malignancy, this condition is termed simple nodular goiter.[32] The pathogenesis of simple nodular goiter is related to genetic and environmental factors, most importantly iodine deficiency. To compensate for inadequate thyroid hormone output, follicular epithelium undergoes compensatory hypertrophy to achieve a euthyroid state. Hypo- or hyperthyroidism may develop. Initially, the goiterous enlargement is diffuse. However, with time it usually becomes nodular. If the impediment to thyroid hormone output abates, the thyroid gland may revert to normal during the diffuse state.

Diffuse nontoxic goiter represents diffuse, nonnodular enlargement of the thyroid associated with a euthyroid state. There are two stages. The first is hyperplasia (follicular cell growth) characterized by diffuse glandular enlargement and hyperemia. The second stage is colloid involution, which occurs when a euthyroid state is maintained. Endemic goiters are prevalent in iodine-deficient areas. There is a female predominance and a peak incidence at puberty.[14] Most simple goiters progress to multinodular goiter that may remain nontoxic and are characterized by nodularity, focal hemorrhage, focal calcifications, and cyst formation. Glandular enlargement may be asymmetric, involving one lobe more than the other, or the isthmus. Thyroid goiters may extend substernally into the anterior mediastinum. A solitary cold nodule in a multinodular gland has similar cancer rates as those of a solitary cold nodule in a normal gland.[33–35] Therefore, a dominant or enlarging mass within a goiterous thyroid raises concern for a malignancy and should be histologically sampled.[36]

Sonography is often able to differentiate among the various causes of an enlarged thyroid gland.

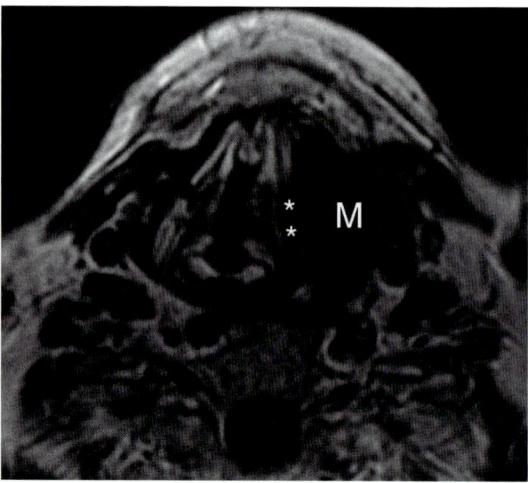

Fig. 3. Tall-cell variant papillary cancer invading the adjacent soft tissues of the neck. Axial T1-W MR image shows the cancer (*M*) in the left lobe of the thyroid gland with poorly demarcated margins and extension into the adjacent carotid space and overlying muscles. Also note invasion of the left thyroid cartilage (*double asterisks*).

On ultrasound, CT, or MR imaging, multinodular goiter has multiple nodules of varying size. These nodules commonly contain complex cystic areas, representing colloid often mixed with areas of hemorrhage and necrosis. Dystrophic calcifications are common and typically are coarse and large. On T1-W MR images, foci of high signal intensity may represent cysts with colloid or hemorrhage. On T2-W MR images, diffuse heterogeneity may be present,[37] and nodules as small as 3 to 5 mm can be visualized.[27] Unlike ultrasound and CT, calcifications may be difficult to detect on MR imaging.

CT and MR imaging are the most valuable imaging modalities in assessing secondary manifestations of goiter, including compression and displacement of the trachea, esophagus, and adjacent vessels (**Fig. 4**). Substernal and mediastinal extension are readily detected. When symptoms related to compression of the aerodigestive tract or vessels occur in elderly patients, nonsurgical candidates, or those refusing surgery, therapy with I-131 may be effective in reducing thyroid volume.[32,38]

Benign Adenomas

Thyroid adenomas are true benign neoplasms distinct from adjacent thyroid tissue and encased by a fibrous capsule. They are usually solitary and nonfunctioning, often detected in young and middle-aged adults. Autonomously functioning adenomas less than 3 mm in diameter are usually not associated with hyperthyroidism.[39] Toxicity is usually associated with large lesions and advanced age. Follicular adenomas slowly increase in size, usually not exceeding 4 cm in diameter.[14] Sudden enlargement of a follicular adenoma is usually related to spontaneous hemorrhage within the lesion.[40] Most thyroid cysts represent spontaneous degeneration of adenomas. Carcinoma within an adenoma is exceedingly rare.[40]

If an adenoma is autonomous (independent of thyrotropin), ablation with I-131 may be performed, as the short-acting beta-radiation will deposit preferentially in the nodule. Alternatively, the nodule may be surgically removed. The previously suppressed normal thyroid tissue resumes normal function following treatment. The risk of postprocedural hypothyroidism is small. Ethanol injection, including with ultrasound guidance, has been reported. However, it has not gained wide acceptance.[41–49]

Evaluation of Thyroid Nodules that are Cancer

Thyroid nodules are common, with palpable nodules occurring in 4% to 7% of the adult population in the United States.[50] Fine needle aspiration of all palpable nodules to assess for cancer in euthyroid patients is the accepted standard of care. In the hands of experienced cytologists, fine needle aspiration has a high accuracy rate.[50] Several factors influence the likelihood that a nodule is cancer. Malignancy is more common in patients under 20 or over 60 years of age, and is more common in men. Findings on physical examination associated with an increased risk of malignancy include firmness of the nodule, rapid growth, fixation to adjacent structures, vocal cord paralysis, and enlarged cervical lymph nodes. A history of neck irradiation or a family history of thyroid cancer also increases the risk that a nodule is cancer.[17,43,44]

The purpose of CT and MR imaging in assessing patients with a suspected thyroid malignancy is to evaluate for extension of tumor outside the thyroid capsule and into adjacent soft tissues of the neck. This should be suspected in patients with complicated clinical presentations (see below). In certain circumstances, CT and MR imaging are also important in assessing for cervical and mediastinal lymph nodal metastases, especially when there is adenopathy on clinical examination as imaging will help determine the extent and type of neck dissection.

MALIGNANT NEOPLASMS OF THE THYROID GLAND

The incidence of thyroid cancer increased up through 1975. This increase, many believe,

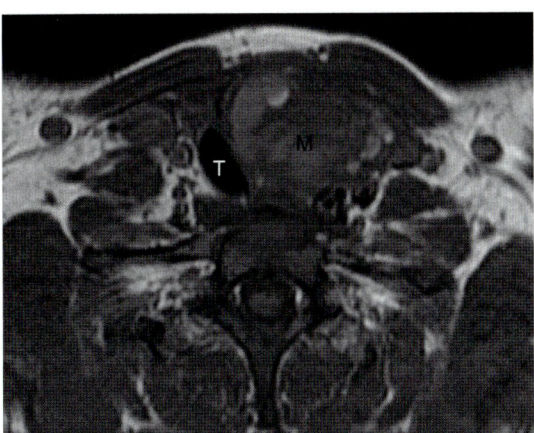

Fig. 4. Thirty-five-year-old woman with palpable left thyroid enlargement. Axial T1-W MR image shows a large mass (*M*) in the left lobe of the thyroid gland, which compresses the trachea (*T*), which is displaced from left to right. Also note there is about 30% luminal narrowing of the trachea.

stemmed from the use for years of low-dose radiation to treat children for benign diseases, especially conditions of the head and neck, such as thymic enlargement and adenoidal hypertrophy.[51] There is a linear dose–response relationship between 100 and 2000 rads.[17,52] Approximately 6% to 8% of patients who receive radiation in this dose range develop papillary thyroid cancer. Long-term follow-up is necessary because the latent period for the development of cancer may be as long as 30 years. Thyroid carcinoma following high-dose irradiation (>2000 rad) is rare, likely because radiation at these doses destroys thyroid tissue.[17] Each year, 20,000 to 30,000 new cases of thyroid carcinoma are diagnosed in the United States. The annual death toll is approximately 1500.[53] The prevalence of incidental thyroid carcinomas identified at autopsy is as high as 18%,[53] and at surgery 10.5%.[54]

Thyroid carcinomas arise from both follicular and parafollicular C-cells. Differentiated carcinomas include papillary and follicular subtypes, which have a favorable prognosis and account for the majority of thyroid cancers.[17,55] Malignant potential and behavior ranges from low-grade (papillary carcinoma) to aggressive (anaplastic carcinoma) and is reflected by mortality rates: papillary carcinoma 8% to 11%, follicular carcinoma 24% to 33%, medullary carcinoma 50%, and anaplastic carcinoma 75% to 90%.[43] Gender, biological behavior, tumor size, and the tendency for hematogenous or lymphatic metastases affect prognosis.

Papillary Carcinoma

Papillary carcinoma is a low-grade malignancy occurring most often in female adolescents and young adults. It comprises up to 80% of thyroid cancers. Histologically, papillary carcinoma may be purely papillary, mixed papillary and follicular, or purely follicular.[56–58] The mixed papillary and completely follicular variants are also included under papillary carcinomas because both biologically and clinically they behave like these tumors.[1,56] Frequently, papillary carcinoma is multifocal in the thyroid gland felt to represent intraglandular lymphatic spread rather than multiple synchronous tumors. Other common patterns of papillary cancer include occult cancers (<1.5 cm in diameter), intrathyroidal encapsulated, and extrathyroidal.[59,60] At gross pathology, these tumors may have calcium, hemorrhage, necrosis, or cysts. Histologically, papillary cancer is characterized by the presence of papillae (epithelial cells encasing a fibrovascular core), and clear nuclei.[57,58] Psammoma bodies (calcified remnants of papillae) are present in over one third of papillary cancers.

There are histologic subtypes of papillary cancer that behave more aggressively, including tall-cell and columnar-cell variants.[61] The tall-cell variant is composed of oxyphilic (pink) cells.[61] At presentation, these variants have a higher incidence of extrathyroidal extension, with vascular or laryngeal invasion, and have a poorer prognosis compared with other papillary carcinomas (see **Fig. 4**).

Papillary carcinoma has the highest incidence of the thyroid malignancies for cervical lymph node metastases, seen in up to 50% of cases. Metastatic lymph nodes are frequently normal in size and may be calcified, vascular, cystic, or hemorrhagic, or they may contain colloid.[62] Thyroglobulin- and colloid-containing metastatic lymph nodes may be hyperintense relative to the neck muscles on unenhanced T1-W MR images (**Fig. 5**), and may have hemorrhage-fluid levels. The differing signal characteristics of complex fluid

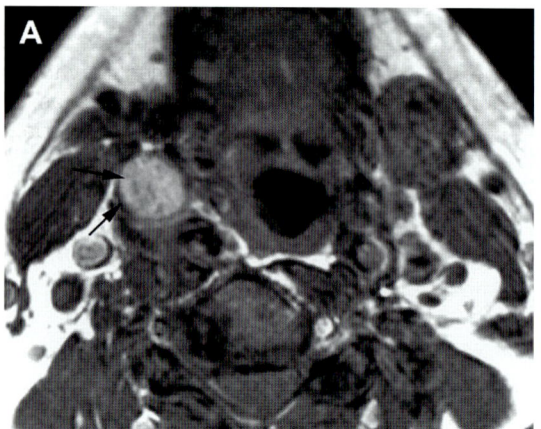 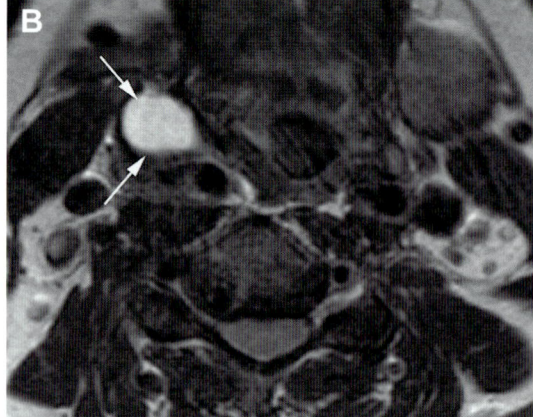

Fig. 5. Papillary thyroid carcinoma with lymph node metastasis. Axial unenhanced T1-W MR image (*A*) shows a hyperintense node in the right level II (*arrows*) pathologically proven to be papillary thyroid cancer metastasis. Axial T2-W MR image (*B*) shows that the cystic node (*arrows*) is hyperintense.

on T1-W and T2-W MR images reflect viscosity, protein concentration, cross-linking of glycoproteins, and water content. Though the vast majority of nodal metastases from thyroid cancer occur in the lateral cervical lymph chains and less commonly in the upper mediastinum, occasionally (2%) metastases occur in retropharyngeal nodes (**Fig. 6**).

Hematogenous spread to the lungs, bones, and central nervous system may occur. However, this is less common (approximately 5%), especially in the absence of nodal disease. Because many papillary carcinomas concentrate radioiodine, scanning with I-131 following thyroidectomy is valuable in identifying recurrent or residual thyroid disease in the operative bed of the neck as well as in detecting cervical and distant metastases. Treatment subsequently with I-131 may be performed. The prognosis for papillary thyroid carcinoma is excellent, with a 20-year survival rate of over 90%.[56–60]

Follicular Carcinoma

True follicular carcinomas constitute 5% of thyroid cancers. They are well-differentiated, relatively low-grade malignancies that are more common in the setting of iodine deficiency. They are slightly more aggressive than papillary carcinomas if vascular invasion is present. Pathologically, they are characterized by capsular and vascular invasion, and are usually solitary. Distant metastases to the lung and bone from hematogenous spread are more common than lymph node metastases, which are seen in less than 8% to 10% of cases.[63] The 5-year survival rate for encapsulated tumors is approximately 90%. However, invasive tumors have a poorer prognosis. Follicular cancers concentrate iodine and I-131 imaging may be useful in the evaluation and follow-up of these patients.

Hürthle-Cell Tumor

Hürthle cells are derived from follicular epithelium and must meet specific criteria. For example, they must be part of an isolated thyroid mass composed predominantly of Hürthle cells and in the absence of inflammatory cells.[64,65] These tumors are diagnosed according to the criterion of malignancy used for follicular neoplasms of the thyroid gland. Regional nodal metastases, in addition to hematogenous dissemination, may occur.

Medullary Carcinoma

Medullary carcinoma is uncommon and has a higher mortality rate than that of differentiated thyroid malignancies. Sporadic medullary carcinomas are usually solitary lesions. They may invade adjacent tissues in the neck, spread to cervical lymph nodes,[66] and spread hematogenously with distant metastases, most commonly to the lungs, bones, and liver. Because of their origin from parafollicular C-cells that secrete calcitonin (up to 90% of medullary carcinomas secrete calcitonin), calcitonin is an excellent hormonal marker for following these patients.[67,68]

Medullary carcinoma may also be inherited in an autosomal dominant pattern (approximately 15% are familial) and comprises a component of the multiple endocrine neoplasia (MEN) syndromes, types IIA and IIB, which include medullary thyroid carcinoma and adrenal pheochromocytomas.[69,70] Hyperparathyroidism is common in MEN type IIA (Sipple's syndrome) due to hyperplasia of the parathyroid glands.[69,70]

Medullary carcinomas may be encapsulated or infiltrative on gross pathology.[69,70] There is a broad spectrum of histologic and biochemical subtypes. The prognosis is variable. Patients with medullary thyroid cancer in the setting of MEN type IIB tend to have very aggressive, often fatal tumors that frequently occur at a young age, while those in association with MEN type IIA have more favorable outcomes.[71] Sporadic tumors may behave in an indolent manner, or may be aggressive.[71] Serum levels of calcitonin and carcinoembryonic

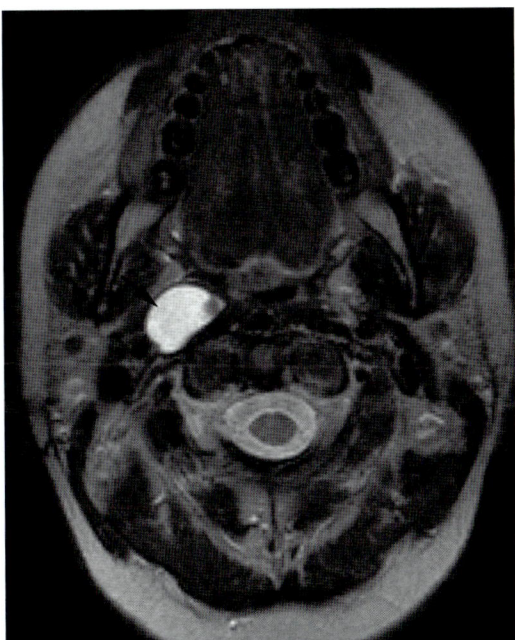

Fig. 6. Twenty-eight-year-old woman with retropharyngeal lymph node metastasis. Axial T2-W MR image shows a cystic right retropharyngeal lymph node metastasis (*arrow*).

antigen, as well as immunostaining of resected tumor, may help predict tumor behavior.[72]

Medullary carcinoma does not concentrate radioiodine. However, radionuclides specific for neuroendocrine tissue, such as I-131 meta-iodobenzylguanidine and the somatostatin analog indium 111 pentetreotide, have been used with some success to evaluate primary as well as metastatic medullary thyroid carcinoma.[73–76]

Anaplastic Carcinoma

Anaplastic carcinoma usually presents in older patients and is highly aggressive and rapidly fatal. Life expectancy is measured in months. It commonly occurs in patients with long-standing goiter. These cancers grow rapidly and typically compress and invade the aerodigestive tract and vessels.[31,66,67,77] Lymph node metastases occur in the majority of patients and are necrotic in approximately 50% of cases.[67,78] Anaplastic carcinomas do not concentrate radioiodine.

Rare Malignancies Affecting Thyroid Gland

Primary lymphoma of the thyroid gland is uncommon and usually presents in elderly women with a long history of goiter. Patients with Hashimoto's thyroiditis also have an increased incidence of thyroid lymphoma, which is usually non-Hodgkin in nature.[79,80] Imaging, including MR, cannot reliably distinguish lymphoma from thyroiditis in patients with Hashimoto's.[13,81] Patients usually present with a rapidly enlarging thyroid mass and obstructive symptoms related to compression of the aerodigestive tract.[13,79] Thyroid lymphoma may present as multiple nodules, but 80% present as a solitary mass.[13,79]

Primary squamous cell carcinoma of the thyroid gland is rare and may result from squamous metaplasia of epithelial cells. Rare sporadic cases of mucoepidermoid carcinoma have been reported. These are typically seen in patients with a long history of goiter and have a poor prognosis. Primary sarcomas of the thyroid gland are extremely rare, may be radiation-induced, and have a poor prognosis.

Metastatic disease to the thyroid gland is rare. Lung and breast carcinoma are the most common metastases found at autopsy, while renal carcinoma is the most common metastasis reported clinically.[82] Metastatic melanoma and colon carcinoma to the thyroid gland have also been reported.[83] Single or multiple thyroid masses may be present in the setting of metastatic disease. When atypical histology of a resected thyroid mass is detected, metastatic disease should be considered. Testing to establish the presence of thyroglobulin or calcitonin supporting that the neoplasm is thyroid in origin may be extremely useful. The absence of these markers favors metastatic disease.

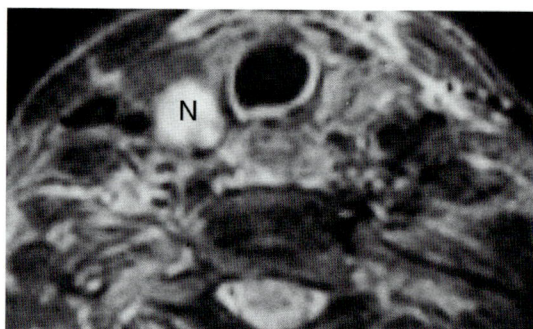

Fig. 7. Benign nodule in goiter. Axial gadolinium-enhanced T1-W MR image shows a patient with underlying goiter and a dominant solidly enhancing nodule (N) in the right lobe of the thyroid gland, which represented a hyperplastic nodule.

THE ROLE OF THE RADIOLOGIST IN THE EVALUATION OF THYROID CANCER
At Initial Clinical Presentation

This section addresses the issue of when to perform cross-sectional imaging in the setting of newly diagnosed differentiated thyroid cancer, including indications for CT or MR imaging of the primary thyroid neoplasm, as well as when to use these modalities in assessing regional nodal metastases. The role of the radiologist in the assessment of patients presenting with thyroid cancer is twofold: (1) to determine the extent of the primary thyroid cancer, and (2) to evaluate for cervical nodal metastases. The less common, more

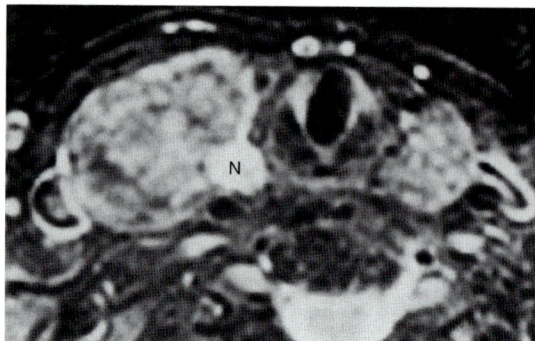

Fig. 8. Cancer in goiter. Axial gadolinium-enhanced T1-W MR image shows a patient with underlying goiter and a dominant solidly enhancing nodule (N) in the right lobe of the thyroid gland, which represented follicular carcinoma at surgery. Note the overall similar appearance to the patient in **Fig. 7**.

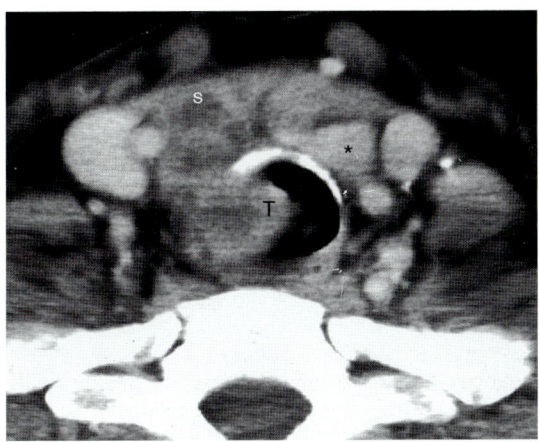

Fig. 9. Forty-eight-year-old patient with tall-cell variant papillary cancer and progressive dyspnea. Axial enhanced CT image obtained to evaluate the patient's respiratory symptoms shows a mass in the inferior right thyroid lobe with extracapsular extension into the strap muscles (S), and gross extension into the trachea (T). Asterisk indicates normal left lobe of thyroid gland.

aggressive cancers usually undergo CT or MR imaging as part of their routine evaluation.

If the initial clinical presentation of a differentiated thyroid cancer is uncomplicated, namely, (1) an isolated asymptomatic thyroid mass detected because it is palpable or because it is incidentally noted on imaging being performed for other reasons, and (2) there is no associated palpable lateral neck adenopathy, all that may be needed is thyroid ultrasound. Ultrasound should be the primary imaging modality in assessing uncomplicated thyroid nodules for several reasons, including its ready availability, its low cost, its superiority to CT or MR imaging in characterizing internal features of a thyroid nodule that may be suspicious for malignancy, and its suitability for fine needle aspiration of concerning nodules under ultrasound guidance (see **Fig. 2**). The main role of CT and MR imaging is not in the characterization of contained intrathyroidal nodules because no imaging findings using these modalities are histologically specific. Benign and malignant nodules may have similar imaging appearances (**Figs. 7** and **8**). It is not uncommon for the neck to be clinically negative despite the presence of metastatic disease in cervical lymph nodes (up to 65% of cancer-harboring nodes in thyroid cancer are normal in size at pathology). In these cases and in the hands of skilled clinicians, imaging outside of ultrasound may not be necessary because nodes with microscopic cancer are treated with iodine radioablation following thyroidectomy. In the minority of patients with noniodine avid tumors at presentation, imaging may be performed to plan the type of neck dissection.

There are specific symptoms associated with thyroid masses that necessitate imaging as part of their evaluation. If the patient presents with a fixed, immobile thyroid mass or is symptomatic with hoarseness, dysphagia, or respiratory symptoms, CT or MR imaging should be obtained. These symptoms are worrisome for spread of neoplasm outside the thyroid capsule. The role of cross-sectional imaging is to identify issues that

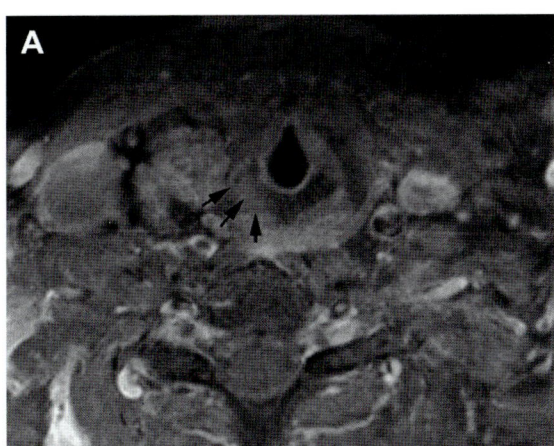 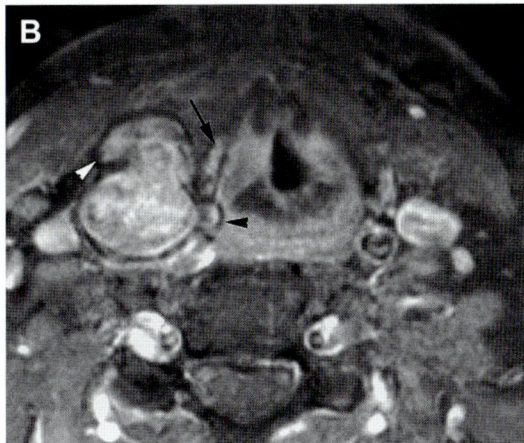

Fig. 10. Fifty-six-year-old woman with extracapsular spread and laryngeal invasion from papillary thyroid cancer. (A) Axial postgadolinium fat-saturated T1-W MR image shows, in the right thyroid lobe, an enhancing mass that invades the right cricoid cartilage (arrows). Note the normal hypointense suppressed fat in the left aspect of the cricoid cartilage. (B) Axial postgadolimium fat-saturated T1-W MR image shows enhancement in the right thyroid cartilage (black arrow) and extension through the cricothyroid membrane (black arrowhead). Extracapsular spread into perithyroidal tissues is present (white arrowhead). Findings were confirmed at surgery.

affect prognosis and allow the surgeon to plan the extent of surgery, and to provide the information necessary to counsel patients preoperatively regarding what to expect in the operating room. The radiologist must determine the extent of the primary tumor, including the identification of the following: (1) spread outside the thyroid capsule to the anterior soft tissues of the neck (strap muscles, sternocleidomastoid muscle) (**Fig. 9**); (2) spread to the airway (larynx or trachea) (see **Fig. 9**; **Fig. 10**); (3) esophageal invasion and, on rare occasions, (4) vascular invasion (**Fig. 11**); (5) spread to the prevertebral muscles or bone (**Fig. 12**); and (6) mediastinal extension. Extension of neoplasm to these locations may necessitate planned combined procedures with thoracic surgery. In certain circumstances, the patient may not be considered a surgical candidate.

In the setting of palpable cervical nodal disease, imaging is frequently requested by the surgeon to plan the extent of neck dissection, and to evaluate the contralateral neck and central compartment and mediastinum for surgical planning. Lymphatic metastatic routes from the thyroid gland include (1) inferiorly to recurrent laryngeal nodes, ventral and lateral tracheal nodes, and superior mediastinal nodes; (2) superiorly to prelaryngeal and paraglandular nodes, and to upper jugular cervical nodes; (3) laterally to lower and midjugular cervical nodes; and (4) posteriorly to retropharyngeal and retroesophageal nodes. The posterior lymphatic drainage is especially important in the thyroidectomy patient being assessed for recurrence. While cervical nodal metastases are frequently of normal size, many of the nodes have abnormal architecture, making them detectable on imaging. Nodal metastases may be solid, cystic (**Fig. 13**), or calcified. In addition, because many nodal metastases may contain colloid, thyroglobulin, or blood products, they may be hyperdense on unenhanced CT, and hyperintense on unenhanced T1-W MR

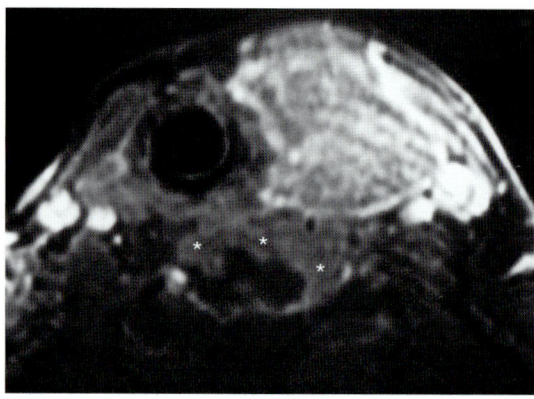

Fig. 12. Patient presented with fixed left neck mass and pain. Axial gadolinium-enhanced fat-saturated T1-W MR image shows a large mass of the left thyroid lobe with posterior extracapsular extension into the prevertebral muscles and encasement of the vertebral body (*asterisks*). Subsequent fine needle aspiration confirmed medullary carcinoma.

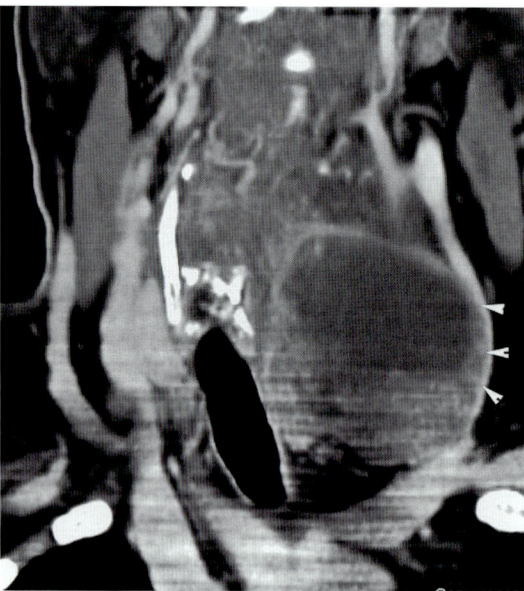

Fig. 11. Forty-five-year-old male presented with a fixed left neck mass. Coronal enhanced CT image shows a large left thyroid lobe mass with surgically confirmed invasion of the perithyroidal tissues, including the internal jugular vein (*arrowheads*). Invasion of the superficial layer of the esophagus was also confirmed at surgery.

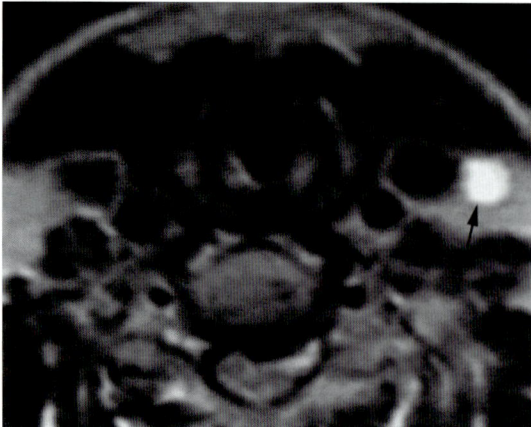

Fig. 13. Normal-size metastatic cystic node. Axial T2-W fat-saturated MR image of the neck in a 27-year-old woman with known papillary thyroid cancer demonstrates a normal-size cystic node (6 mm) in the left level III (*arrow*). This node was nonpalpable.

images (see **Fig. 5**), making them identifiable with careful image analysis.

Imaging the Treated Neck with Rising Thyroglobulin

Following thyroidectomy for differentiated thyroid cancer, serum thyroglobulin is an excellent marker to detect the presence of recurrent cancer. One of the most significant dilemmas clinicians face is in detecting the site of recurrence in patients following thyroidectomy with rising thyroglobulin and normal clinical examination (no palpable disease). Recurrent disease is frequently within cervical lymph nodes, but less commonly may represent distant metastases to the lungs, bones, and occasionally the brain. The role of imaging in the setting of the treated neck with rising thyroglobulin is to identify clinically occult metastases.

Imaging in recurrent disease may include ultrasound of the lateral neck with fine needle aspiration as required, cross-sectional imaging (CT or MR), I-131 whole-body scan, and/or PET–CT.[24,84–86] Ultrasound is sensitive in detecting cancer in lateral cervical lymph nodes that are normal in size as it readily detects abnormal echogenicity and blood flow in them, but it has low accuracy in assessing the deep spaces of the head and neck (retropharyngeal nodes and mediastinum), which are the strengths of CT and MR imaging (see **Fig. 6**; **Fig. 14**). Diagnostic CT often requires iodinated contrast that may be contraindicated if I-131 whole-body scanning or radioablation therapy is a consideration. Whole-body I-131 imaging is most accurate in detecting iodine avid metastases, but can miss up to 50% of differentiated/dedifferentiated thyroid metastases. In patients with thyroid cancer, whole-body I-131 scanning has an overall sensitivity of approximately 50%, and specificity over 95%.[84] It my may require withdrawal of thyroid hormone therapy or the administration of thyroid stimulating hormone. Advantages of MR imaging in detecting metastases is that there are no concerns about iodinated contrast agents. In addition, lymph nodes harboring metastatic thyroid cancer frequently have high protein content due to the presence of thyroglobulin, colloid, and occasionally blood products, making them detectable on MR imaging ("bright" hyperintense on unenhanced T1-W imaging). MR imaging is 90% to 95% sensitive when thyroglobulin is elevated. In patients in whom MR or CT identifies nodes suspected of harboring cancer, CT-guided fine needle aspiration can readily be performed for histologic confirmation (**Fig. 15**).

The role of PET or PET–CT in the assessment of differentiated thyroid cancer recurrence is still evolving. The uptake of FDG in general is inversely proportional to iodine uptake/differentiation.[85] Its overall sensitivity is approximately 65% (iodine avid 50%–65%, noniodine avid 70%–85%).[24,84,85] Its overall specificity is greater than 95%.[85] Another limitation of PET is that cancerous nodes may not be detected on PET due to low cellularity, or because they are predominantly cystic or necrotic. In addition, even noniodine avid

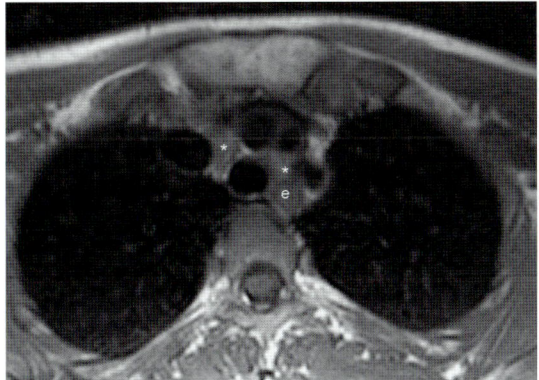

Fig. 14. Recurrent papillary carcinoma in patient with rising thyroglobulin and negative neck ultrasound. Axial T1-W MR image shows multiple metastatic lymph nodes in the superior mediastinum (*asterisks*) that are mildly hyperintense. (e) Esophagus.

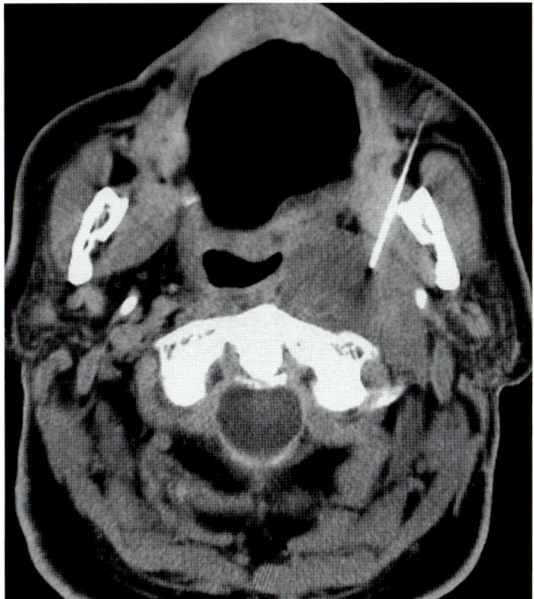

Fig. 15. Recurrent papillary cancer at the skull base. Axial unenhanced CT image shows a large mass at the left base of skull with CT-guided needle positioned within it to get a tissue sample. Fine needle aspiration revealed recurrent papillary cancer with anaplastic transformation.

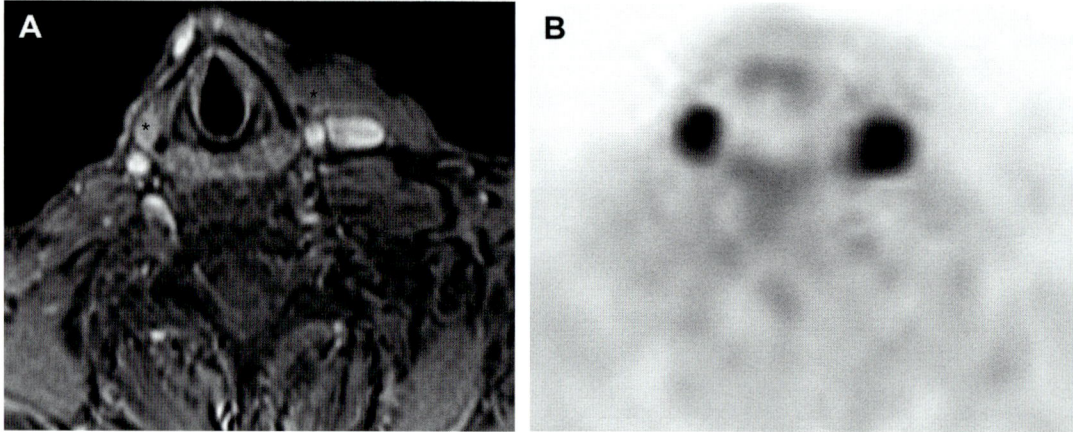

Fig. 16. Recurrent papillary cancer. (A) Axial fat-saturated gadolinium-enhanced T1-W MR image shows a small nodule anterior to the right common carotid artery along the right thyroid cartilage (*left asterisk*), as well as anterior to the left carotid sheath (*right asterisk*). (B) FDG PET shows avid uptake in these small suspicious areas seen on MR image, consistent with recurrence.

small metastases, such as those in the lungs, may be missed because of low cellularity. Some clinicians see an additional role of PET–CT in the evaluation of recurrent papillary cancer. They say that PET–CT may provide additional information that confirms or changes the management plan, and enhances patient and physician confidence in both the diagnosis of metastatic disease (**Fig. 16**) and in the management plan.[85,87] Iodine-based PET agents are in development that will have a significant impact on the role of PET in recurrent thyroid cancer.

In conclusion, recommendations for imaging in the setting of rising thyroglobulin in patients treated for differentiated thyroid cancer with a negative clinical examination should include ultrasound of the thyroid bed and lateral neck, I-131 scan, and MR of the neck and upper mediastinum, and chest CT. In our practice, PET–CT is used when ultrasound, MR, and I-131 scanning are negative or equivocal, as it is in this group that the sensitivity of PET is highest.

THYROGLOSSAL DUCT CYSTS AND CARCINOMA

Incomplete degeneration of the thyroglossal duct may result in a persistent fistulous tract or cyst along the path of migration of the thyroid gland

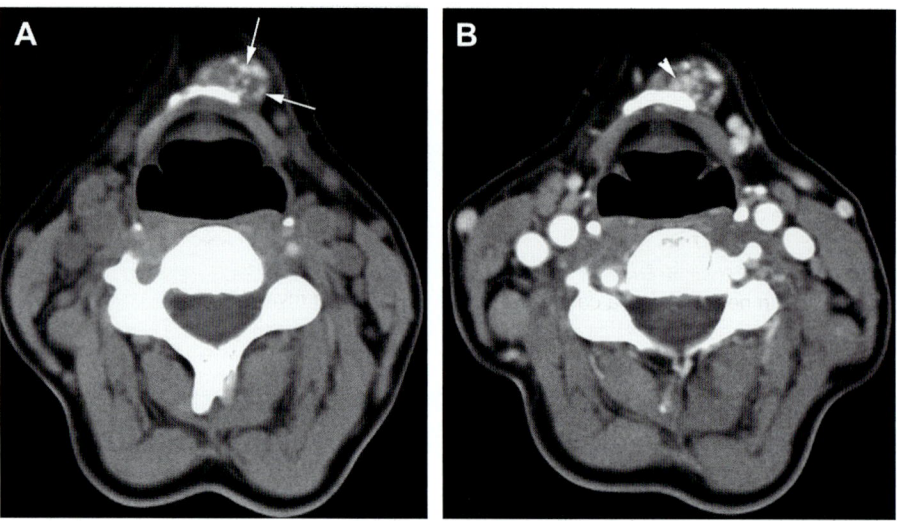

Fig. 17. Forty-nine-year-old woman with an enlarging midline neck mass. (A) Axial unenhanced CT scan shows a heterogeneous predominantly cystic mass embedded in the hyoid bone with multiple calcifications (*arrows*). (B) Contrast-enhanced CT image shows enhancement within the lesion centrally (*arrowhead*). Papillary carcinoma within a thyroglossal duct was confirmed at surgery.

from the foramen cecum at the tongue base to the anterior lower neck. Thyroglossal duct cysts are anterior midline neck masses when they occur at or above the hyoid bone, and tend to be paramedian in location when below the hyoid bone. Over half of these cysts have normal thyroid follicular tissue in their walls.[88] Approximately 65% of thyroglossal duct cysts are infrahyoid in location and are encased by the thyroid strap muscles, 20% of thyroglossal duct cysts are suprahyoid, and 15% of cysts are at the hyoid region above the strap muscles. When large, thyroglossal duct cysts are clinically detected as palpable midline neck masses. Small thyroglossal duct cysts are usually clinically occult and may only be recognized if they become secondarily infected or traumatized, or if they are incidentally noted on imaging studies of the neck being performed for unrelated reasons.

On cross-sectional imaging, uncomplicated thyroglossal duct cysts are usually well demarcated. On MR imaging, they frequently have signal characteristics similar to those of cerebrospinal fluid on T1-W and T2-W images. When the contents of the cyst are proteinaceous, cysts may be hyperintense on T1-W images, and usually remain intermediate-to-hyperintense on T2-W scans. Rarely, thyroglossal duct cysts may undergo malignant degeneration, usually into papillary carcinoma, and this should be suspected when a soft tissue component or nodule exists within or around the cyst (**Fig. 17**), or if the cyst has calcifications.[89]

REFERENCES

1. LiVolsi VA. The thyroid and parathyroid. In: Sternberg SS, editor. Diagnostic surgical pathology. 2nd edition. New York: Raven Press; 1994. p. 523–60.
2. Pintar JE. Toran-Allerand CD: Normal development of the hypothalamic-pituitary-thyroid axis. In: Braverman LE, Utiger RD, editors. Werner and Ingbar's the thyroid. 6th edition. Philadelphia: JB Lippincott Co; 1991. p. 7–21.
3. Morgan NJ, Emberton P, Barton RP. The importance of thyroid scanning in neck lumps—a case report of ectopic tissue in the right submandibular region. J Laryngol Otol 1995;109(7):674–6.
4. Guneri A, Ceryan K, Igci E, et al. Lingual thyroid: the diagnostic value of magnetic resonance imaging. J Laryngol Otol 1991;105(6):493–5.
5. Williams JD, Sclafani AP, Slupchinskij O, et al. Evaluation and management of the lingual thyroid gland. Ann Otol Rhinol Laryngol 1996;105:312–6.
6. Brandwein M, Som P, Urken M. Benign intratracheal thyroid. Arch Otolaryngol Head Neck Surg 1998; 124:1266–9.
7. Kantelip B, Lusson JR, DeRiberolles C, et al. Intracardiac ectopic thyroid. Hum Pathol 1986;17: 1293–6.
8. Fujioka S, Takatsu Y, Tankawa H, et al. Intracardiac ectopic thyroid mass. Chest 1996;110:1366–8.
9. Sandler MP, Patton JA, Ossoff RH. Recent advances in thyroid imaging. Otolaryngol Clin North Am 1990; 23:251–70.
10. Takashima S, Nomura N, Tanaka H, et al. Congenital hypothyroidism: assessment with ultrasound. AJNR Am J Neuroradiol 1995;16(5):1117–23.
11. Shibutani Y, Inoue D, Koshiyama H. Thyroid hemiagenesis with subacute thyroiditis. Thyroid 1995; 5(2):133–5.
12. Ahuja AT, Kind AD, King W, et al. Thyroglossal duct cysts: sonographic appearance in adults. AJNR Am J Neuroradiol 1999;20:579–82.
13. Shibata T, Noma S, Nakano Y, et al. Primary thyroid lymphoma: MR appearance. J Comput Assist Tomogr 1991;15(4):629–33.
14. De Lellis RA. The endocrine system. In: Cotram R, Kumar V, Robbins SL, editors. Robbins pathologic basis of disease. 4th edition. Philadelphia: WB Saunders Co; 1989. p. 1214–42.
15. Plummer HS. The clinical and pathologic relationship of simple and exophthalmic goiter. Am J Med Sci 1913;146:790–803.
16. Villadolid MC, Yokoyama N, Izumi M, et al. Untreated Graves disease patients without clinical ophthalmopathy demonstrate a high frequency of extra-ocular muscle (EOM) enlargement by magnetic resonance. J Clin Endocrinol Metab 1995;80(9):2830–3.
17. Price DC. Radioisotopic evaluation of the thyroid and parathyroids. Radiol Clin North Am 1993;31: 991–1015.
18. Smith JR, Oates E. Radionuclide imaging of the thyroid gland; patterns, pearls and pitfalls. Clin Nucl Med 2004;29:181–93.
19. Nygaard B, Nygaard T, Jensen LI, et al. Iohexol: effects on uptake of radioactive iodine in the thyroid and on thyroid function. Acad Radiol 1998;5:409–14.
20. Laurie AJ, Lyons SG, Lassen EC. Contrast material iodides: potential effects on radioactive thyroid uptake. J Nucl Med 1992;33:237–8.
21. Sternthall E, Lipworth L, Stanley B, et al. Suppression of thyroid radioiodine uptake by various doses of stable iodide. N Engl J Med 1980;303:1083–8.
22. Lauberg P, Boye N. Inhibitory effect of various radiographic contrast agents on secretion of thyroxine by the dog thyroid and on peripheral and thyroidal deiodination of thyroxine to triodothyronine. J Endocrinol 1987;112:387–90.
23. Feine U, Lietzenmayer R, Hanke J, et al. Fluorine-18-FDG and iodine-131 uptake in thyroid cancer. J Nucl Med 1996;37:1468–72.
24. Dietlein M, Scheidhauer K, Voth E, et al. Flourine-18 fluorodeoxyglucose positron emission tomography

and iodine-131 whole body scintigraphy in the follow-up of differentiated thyroid cancer. Eur J Nucl Med 1997;24:1342–8.
25. Wang W, Larson SM, Fazzari M, et al. Prognostic value of [18F] fluorodeoxyglucose positron emission tomographic scanning in patients with thyroid cancer. J Clin Endocrinol Metab 2000;85:1107–13.
26. Gotway MB, Higgins CB. MR imaging of the thyroid and parathyroid glands. Magn Reson Imaging 2000; 8(1):163–82.
27. Gefter W, Spritzer CE, LiVolsi VA, et al. Thyroid imaging with high-field strength surface-coil MR. Radiology 1987;164:483–90.
28. Hopkins CR, Reading CC. Thyroid and parathyroid imaging. Semin Ultrasound CT MR 1995;16(4): 279–95.
29. Quinn SF, Nelson HA, Demlow TA. Thyroid biopsies: fine-needle aspiration biopsy versus spring-activated core biopsy needle in 102 patients. J Vasc Interv Radiol 1994;5(4):619–23.
30. Sanchez RB, vanSonnenberg E, D'Agostino HB, et al. Ultrasound guided biopsy of nonpalpable and difficult to palpate thyroid masses. J Am Coll Surg 1994;178(1):33–7.
31. Hegedus L. Thyroid ultrasound. Endocrinol Metab Clin North Am 2001;30(2):339–60.
32. Langer JE, Khan A, Nisenbaum HL, et al. Sonographic appearance of focal thyroiditis. AJR Am J Roentgenol 2001;176:751–4.
33. Belfiore A, LaRose GL, LaPorta GA, et al. Cancer risks in patients with cold thyroid nodules: relevance of iodine intake, sex, age, and multinodularity. Am J Med 1992;93:363–9.
34. Cerise EJ, Spears R, Ochsner A. Carcinoma of the thyroid and nontoxic nodular goiter. Surgery 1952; 31:552–61.
35. McCall A, Jarosz H, Lawrence AM, et al. The incidence of thyroid carcinoma in solitary cold nodules and in multinodular goiters. Surgery 1986;100: 1128–32.
36. Shulkin BL, Shapiro B. The role of imaging tests in the diagnosis of thyroid carcinoma. Endocrinol Metab Clin North Am 1990;19(3):523–43.
37. Noma S, Kanaoka M, Minami S, et al. Thyroid masses: MR imaging and pathologic correlation. Radiology 1988;168:759–64.
38. Huysmans DA, Hermus AR, Corstens FH, et al. Large, compressive goiters treated with radioiodine. Ann Intern Med 1994;121(10):757–62.
39. Hamberger JI. Evolution of toxicity in solitary nontoxic autonomously functioning thyroid nodules. Clin Endocrinol Metab 1980;50:1089–93.
40. Ross DS. Evaluation of the thyroid nodule. J Nucl Med 1991;32:2181–92.
41. Gharib H, Goellner J. Fine-needle aspiration biopsy of the thyroid: an appraisal. Ann Intern Med 1993; 118:282–9.
42. Yousem DM, Huang T, Loevner LA, et al. Clinical and economic impact of incidental thyroid lesions discovered by CT and MR imaging. AJNR Am J Neuroradiol 1997;18:1423–8.
43. Harvey HK. Diagnosis and management of the thyroid nodule: an overview. Otolaryngol Clin North Am 1990;23:303–37.
44. Hegedus L, Bonnema SJ, Bennedbaek FN. Management of simple nodular goiter: current status and future perspectives. Endocr Rev 2003;24: 102–32.
45. Brander A, Viikinkoski P, Nickels J, et al. Thyroid gland: US screening in a random adult population. Radiology 1991;181:683–7.
46. Bruneton J, Balu-Maestro C, Marcy P, et al. Very high frequency (13MHz) ultrasonographic examination of the normal neck: detection of normal lymph nodes and thyroid nodules. J Ultrasound Med 1994;13: 87–90.
47. Marqusee E, Benson C, Frates M, et al. Usefulness of ultrasonography in the management of nodular thyroid disease. Ann Intern Med 2000;133: 696–700.
48. Valcavi R, Frasoldati A. Ultrasound-guided percutaneous ethanol injection therapy in thyroid cystic nodules. Endocr Pract. 2004;10:269–75.
49. Papini E, Pacella CM, Verde G. Percutaneous ethanol injection (PEI): What is its role in the treatment of benign thyroid nodules? Thyroid 1995; 2:147–50.
50. Dworkin HJ, Meier DA, Kaplan M. Advances in the management of patients with thyroid disease. Semin Nucl Med 1995;5:205–20.
51. Duffy BJ Jr, Fitzgerald PJ. Cancer of the thyroid in children: a report of 28 cases. J Clin Endocrinol Metab 1950;10:1296–311.
52. Favus MJ, Schneider AB, Stachura ME, et al. Thyroid cancer occurring as a late consequence of head-and-neck irradiation: evaluation of 1,056 patients. N Engl J Med 1976;294:1019–25.
53. Mazzaferri EL. Management of a solitary thyroid nodule. N Engl J Med 1993;328:553–9.
54. Pelizzo MR, Piotto A, Rubello D, et al. High prevalence of occult papillary thyroid carcinoma in a surgical series for benign thyroid disease. Tumori 1990;76:255–7.
55. Sutton RT, Reading CC, Charboneau JW, et al. US-guided biopsy of neck masses in postoperative management of patients with thyroid cancer. Radiology 1988;168:769–72.
56. Chen KT, Rosai J. Follicular variant of thyroid papillary carcinoma. A clinicopathologic study of 6 cases. Am J Surg Pathol 1977;1:123–30.
57. Rosai J, Zampi G. Carcangiu. Papillary carcinoma of the thyroid. Am J Surg Pathol 1983;7:809–17.
58. Carcangiu ML, Zampi G, Pupi A, et al. Papillary carcinoma of the thyroid. A clinicopathologic study

59. of 244 cases treated at the University of Florence, Italy. Cancer 1985;55:805–28.
59. Vickery AL. Thyroid papillary carcinoma. Pathological and philosophical controversies. Am J Surg Pathol 1983;7:797–807.
60. Hay ID. Papillary thyroid carcinoma. Endocrinol Metab Clin North Am 1990;19:545–76.
61. Hawk WA, Hazard JB. The many appearances of papillary carcinoma of the thyroid. Cleve Clin Q 1976;43:207–16.
62. Som PM, Brandwein M, Lidov M, et al. The varied appearance of papillary carcinoma cervical nodal disease: CT and MR findings. AJNR Am J Neuroradiol 1994;15:1129–38.
63. Franssila KO, Ackerman LV, Brown CL, et al. Follicular carcinoma. Semin Diagn Pathol 1985;2:101–2.
64. Roediger WE. The oxyphil and C cells of the human thyroid gland. Cancer 1975;36:1758–70.
65. Bondeson L, Bondeson AG, Ljungberg O, et al. Oxyphil tumors of the thyroid. Follow-up of 42 surgical cases. Ann Surg 1981;194:677–80.
66. Gorman B, Charboneau JW, James EM, et al. Medullary thyroid carcinoma: role of high-resolution US. Radiology 1987;162:147–50.
67. Compagno J, Oertel JE. Malignant lymphoma and other lymphoproliferative disorders of the thyroid gland: clinicopathologic study of 245 cases. Am J Clin Pathol 1980;74:1–11.
68. Melvin KE, Miller HH, Tashjian AH. Early diagnosis of medullary carcinoma of the thyroid by means of calcitonin assay. N Engl J Med 1971;285:1115–20.
69. Steiner AL, Goodman AD, Powers SR. Study of a kindred with pheochromocytoma, medullary thyroid carcinoma, hyperparathyroidism, and Cushing's disease: multiple endocrine neoplasia type 2. Medicine 1968;47:371–409.
70. Wolfe HJ, DeLellis RA. Familial medullary thyroid carcinomaand C-cell hyperplasia. Clin Endocrinol Metab 1981;10:351–65.
71. Kakudo K, Carney JA, Sizemore GW. Medullary carcinoma of thyroid: biologic behavior of the sporadic and familial neoplasm. Cancer 1985;55:2818–21.
72. Busnardo B, Girelli ME, Simioni N, et al. Non-parallel patterns of calcitonin and carcinoembryonic antigen levels in the follow-up of medullary thyroid carcinoma. Cancer 1984;53:278–85.
73. Dorr U, Wurstlin S, Frank-Raue K, et al. Somatostatin receptor scintigraphy and magnetic resonance imaging in recurrent medullary thyroid carcinoma: a comparative study. Horm Metab Res Suppl 1993;27:48–55.
74. Lebouthillier G, Morais J, Picard M, et al. Tc-99m sestamibi and other agents in the detection of metastatic medullary carcinoma of the thyroid. Clin Nucl Med 1993;18(8):657–61.
75. Krenning EP, Kwekkeboom DJ, Bakker WH, et al. Somatostatin receptor scintigraphy with [111-In-DTPA-D-phe]- and [I-123-tyr]-octreotide: the Rotterdam experience with more than 1,000 patients. Eur J Nucl Med 1993;20:716–31.
76. Dorr U, Sautter-Bihl ML, Heiner B. The contribution of somatostatin receptor scintigraphy to the diagnosis of recurrent medullary carcinoma of the thyroid. Semin Oncol 1994;21:42–5.
77. Solbiati L, Volterrani L, Rizzatto G, et al. The thyroid gland with low uptake lesions: evaluation by ultrasound. Radiology 1985;155:187–91.
78. Takashima S, Morimoto S, Ikezoe J, et al. CT evaluation of anaplastic thyroid carcinoma. AJR Am J Roentgenol 1990;154:1079–85.
79. Takashima S, Ikezoe J, Morimoto S, et al. Primary thyroid lymphoma: evaluation with CT. Radiology 1988;168:765–8.
80. Ott RA, Calandra DB, McCall A, et al. The incidence of thyroid carcinoma in patients with Hashimoto's thyroiditis and solitary cold nodules. Surgery 1985;98:1202–6.
81. Ohnishi T, Noguchi S, Murakami N, et al. MR imaging in patients with primary thyroid lymphoma. AJNR Am J Neuroradiol 1992;13(4):1196–8.
82. Haugen BR, Nawaz S, Cohn A, et al. Secondary malignancy of the thyroid gland: a case report and review of the literature. Thyroid 1994;4(3):297–300.
83. Czech JM, Lichtor TR, Carney JA, et al. Neoplasms metastatic to the thyroid gland. Surg Gynecol Obstet 1982;155:503–5.
84. Grünwald F, Kalicke T, Feine U, et al. Fluorine-18 fluorodeoxyglucose positron emission tomography in thyroid cancer: results of a multicentre study. Eur J Nucl Med 1999;26:1547–52.
85. Nahas Z, Goldenberg D, Fakhry C, et al. The role of positron emission tomography/computed tomography in the management of recurrent papillary thyroid carcinoma. Laryngoscope 2005;115(2):237–43.
86. Zimmer LA, McCook B, Meltzer C, et al. Combined positron emission tomography/computed tomography imaging of recurrent thyroid cancer. Otolaryngol Head Neck Surg 2003;128:178–84.
87. Frilling A, Tecklenborg K, Gorges R, et al. Preoperative diagnostic value of [18F] fluorodeoxyglucose positron emission tomography in patients with radioiodine-negative recurrent well-differentiated thyroid carcinoma. Ann Surg 2001;234(6):804–11.
88. Pollice L, Caneso G. Struma cordis. Arch Pathol Lab Med 1986;110:452–3.
89. Hays LL, Marlow SF Jr. Papillary carcinoma arising in a thyroglossal duct cyst. Laryngoscope 1968;78:2189–93.

Ultrasound of Thyroid Nodules

Terry S. Desser, MD*, Aya Kamaya, MD

KEYWORDS

- Thyroid nodules • Thyroid carcinoma • Ultrasound
- Sonography

Thyroid nodules are a ubiquitous clinical problem. In years past, when palpation was the sole method of thyroid evaluation, the prevalence of thyroid nodules was estimated at approximately 4% to 8% of the adult population and typically only those nodules 1 cm or larger in diameter were detected.[1] With increasing use of imaging for evaluation of the carotid arteries, cervical spine, and chest, the reported prevalence of thyroid nodules has increased to as high as 40% to 50%,[1–3] approaching the 50% prevalence of nodules found at autopsy. Because the risk for malignancy in these thyroid nodules is low (1.5%–10%), the issue of how best to manage the current epidemic of thyroid nodules in an increasingly cost-constrained environment is a critical one. Furthermore, the vast majority of the cancers detected are papillary carcinomas, which are often clinically occult and virtually never fatal even after spread to regional lymph nodes has occurred.[4–8] A logical strategy for identifying the minority of thyroid nodules that require intervention from among the huge numbers that do not is a topic of much debate among sonographers and endocrinologists.

High-resolution ultrasound is the modality of choice for evaluation of the thyroid gland. It is painless, inexpensive, does not require the use of contrast media, and can display the internal architecture and flow characteristics of nodules as small as 1 to 2 mm. Ultrasound-guided fine-needle aspiration (FNA) with cytologic evaluation is now a mainstay in the management of palpable and incidentally detected nodules. This article reviews the current techniques for sonographic evaluation of the thyroid and the imaging features of the various types of thyroid nodules. We also explore the various strategies for management of thyroid nodules based on clinical and imaging parameters.

ANATOMY AND SCANNING TECHNIQUE

The thyroid gland is an H-shaped organ composed of two lobes joined by a narrow isthmus located just below the laryngeal cartilages. The normal thyroid weighs approximately 15 to 25 g,[9] with each lobe approximately 4 cm in length and 2 cm in thickness. Befitting its vital role in metabolism, it is a highly vascular organ supplied by the superior thyroidal branch of the external carotid artery and the inferior thyroid branch of the subclavian artery. Microscopically, the thyroid parenchyma is organized into follicles, hollow spheres of epithelial cells enclosing a protein-rich material termed colloid. Thin fibrous septations divide the normal thyroid into lobules composed of 20 to 40 follicles each about 50 to 500 μm in size.

To visualize the thyroid gland optimally, the patient is placed in the supine position with a pillow underneath the shoulders to extend the neck slightly, allowing the head to rest on the examination table. In older patients or those who have degenerative changes in the neck, small towels can be placed under the head to the level where the patient is most comfortable while still allowing access to the neck. The thyroid gland is then imaged in transverse and longitudinal views with a high-frequency (10–15 MHz) linear transducer. The highest frequency is used while still allowing adequate sonographic penetration.

The normal thyroid gland is uniformly echogenic relative to the overlying strap muscles of the neck (**Fig. 1**). A thyroid nodule is defined as a region of

---

Department of Radiology, Stanford University School of Medicine, 300 Pasteur Drive, Mail Code 5621, Stanford, CA 94305, USA
* Corresponding author.
E-mail address: desser@stanford.edu (T.S. Desser).

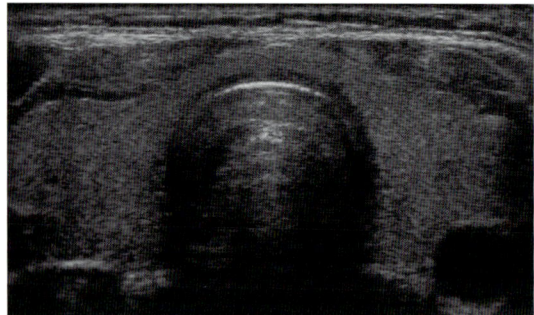

Fig. 1. Transverse gray-scale mode image of a normal thyroid gland, which is uniformly echogenic relative to overlying strap musculature.

parenchyma sonographically distinct from the remainder of the thyroid and located within the confines of the echogenic thyroid capsule. When a nodule is detected, its size should be measured in three dimensions and the location within the thyroid gland (upper pole, mid-gland, lower pole) should be noted by the sonographer. Several sonographic features are helpful for differential diagnosis, including nodule echogenicity, morphology, cystic change, presence of echogenic foci with comet-tail artifact representing colloid, presence and type of calcifications, and flow pattern (peripheral or central). These are discussed in more detail later.

Instrumentation: New Technologies

Several new sonographic technologies have been applied to the imaging of thyroid nodules. Three-dimensional (3D) ultrasound, in which a free-hand or automated sweep of the transducer generates an image volume that can be displayed in axial, coronal, or sagittal planes, can generate good-quality images of multinodular thyroids (**Fig. 2**). In a recent study comparing volume measurements of thyroid nodules in 102 children, 3D ultrasound measurements were more accurate, with less intraobserver variability and higher reproducibility, compared with two-dimensional assessment.[10] It may also provide greater workflow efficiency, because entire organs can be scanned in a single transducer sweep.[11] Compound imaging is a signal-averaging technique designed to reduce speckle noise and improve contrast resolution, and has been shown to increase contrast-to-noise ratio in clinical thyroid images (**Fig. 3**).[12] Tissue harmonic imaging (THI) uses the first harmonic of the transmitted frequency for

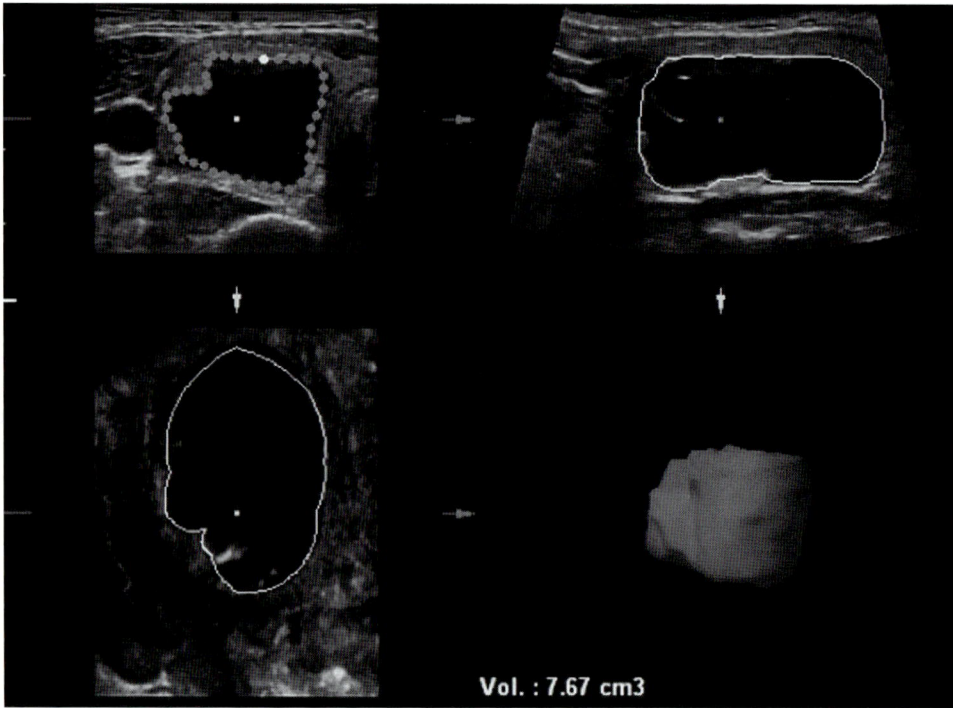

Fig. 2. Volumetric display of cystic thyroid nodule with calculation of nodule volume. A single sweep through the image volume is obtained, and three orthogonal planes are displayed. Upper left image is axial plane, upper right image is sagittal plane, and lower left image is coronal plane. Lower right image shows volume rendering of cystic nodule, with calculated volume beneath. (*Courtesy of* GE Healthcare Technologies.)

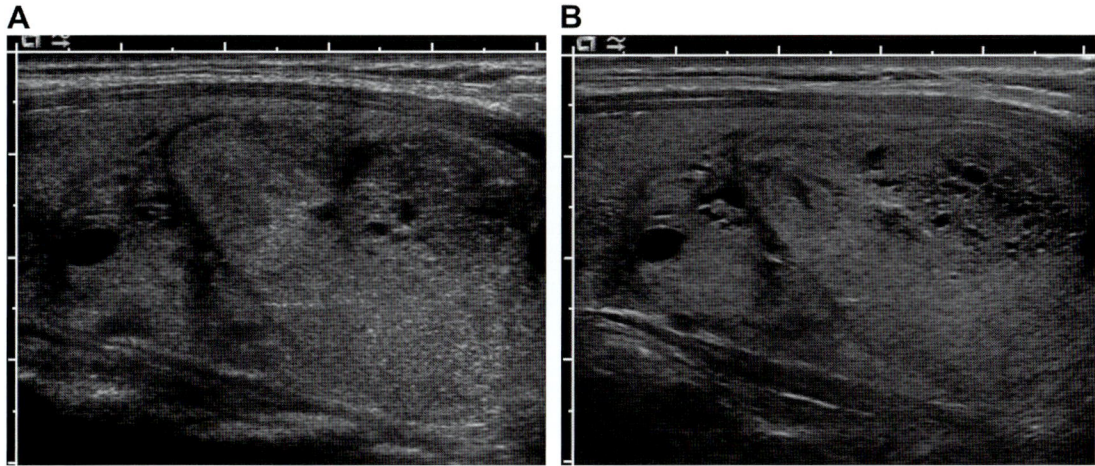

Fig. 3. Sagittal images of complex solid and cystic thyroid nodule. (A) Image obtained with conventional high-resolution transducer shows small cystic areas in lower portion of nodule. (B) Image obtained at higher frequency and with compounding shows better spatial resolution of tiny cystic areas. (*Courtesy of* Siemens Medical Systems.)

image formation and results in images with less noise. Its benefits in abdominal and pelvic sonography are dramatic, especially in obese patients. In a study of 144 patients who had thyroid nodules, THI improved lesion conspicuity and gray-scale contrast between lesions;[13] however, the fundamental mode imaging was performed at 7.5 MHz, and therefore the relevance of this work is questionable given that most thyroid ultrasound is performed at 10 MHz or higher. Although these innovations have improved image clarity somewhat, they have not impacted lesion characterization significantly. Similarly, sonographic contrast agents have been used in other organ systems, but to date have not had a significant role in thyroid nodule imaging.

Elastography

By contrast, elastography of thyroid nodules is an evolving technology with early reported promise of differentiating benign nodules from malignant nodules with 96% specificity and 82% specificity.[14] Analogous to palpation, the rationale behind elastography is that a cancerous nodule is stiffer, with less elastic deformation compared with muscle or a benign thyroid nodule. Ultrasound elastography is a dynamic method in which an external compressive force is applied during scanning and the degree of distortion used to estimate the stiffness of the tissue of interest (**Fig. 4**). Ultrasound elastography has already been used to differentiate cancer from benign lesions in the prostate, breast, pancreas, and lymph nodes.[15] Different methods of identifying a stiff thyroid nodule are currently being studied, including manual compression with comparison of the lesion during a cine loop using speckle tracking in two and three dimensions, or with evaluation of the nodule under normal respiratory and cardiac pulsations. One recent study used carotid artery pulsation as the compression source and found that elastography was able to distinguish a papillary carcinoma from a benign nodule located in the same thyroid lobe.[16] Although these implementations of elastography require off-line image processing, some newer machines are capable of real-time image processing. Recent work using a real-time elastography technique in 92 consecutive patients who had solitary thyroid nodules found that elastography scores representing the least strain (stiff lesions with little deformation) were highly predictive of malignancy with sensitivity of 97%, specificity of 100%, and 100% positive predictive value.[15] The patients were highly selected, however, and cystic nodules, nodules with eggshell calcification, and patients who had multiple nodules were not included in the study. Although promising, elastography needs further study to determine whether the method will prove as robust when used on a larger scale.

THYROID NODULES

Various benign and malignant nodules occur commonly in the thyroid gland (**Box 1**). In the Framingham population study, nodules were found by palpation in 6.4% of women and 1.5% of men.[8] By ultrasound, many more nodules are detected. In one study, 50% of patients who had apparent solitary nodules by palpation had additional nodules detected by ultrasound, and about 25% of those nodules were larger than 1 cm.[17] Location

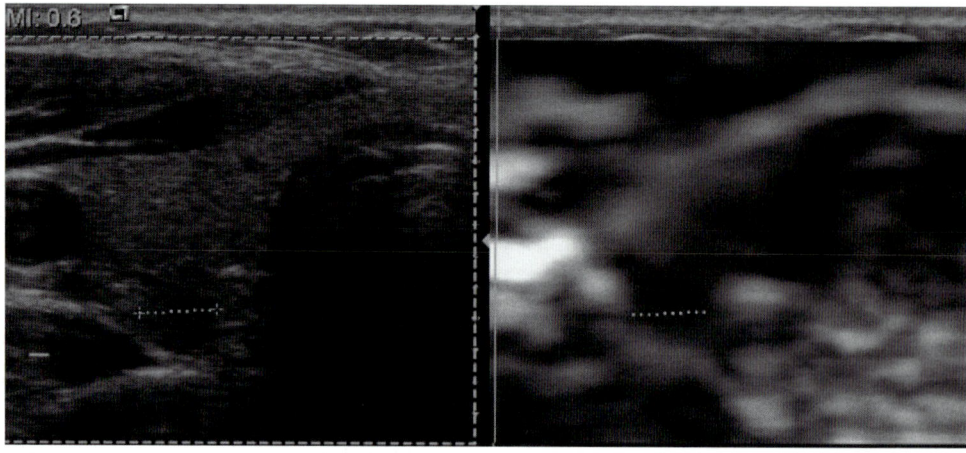

Fig. 4. Simultaneous gray-scale and elastography image of a biopsy-proven benign thyroid nodule. Image on left is a gray-scale image of a thyroid nodule demarcated by calipers. Image on right is corresponding elastography image at same location. On elastography image, the nodule (dark area behind calipers) is smaller in size compared with the nodule seen on gray-scale, which suggests this lesion is more compressible than the adjacent thyroid parenchyma. This finding correlates with a benign pathology.

of the nodule (anterior or posterior), size of the patient's neck, and skill of the examiner all affect the likelihood of detection by palpation. With current ultrasound technology, however, even nodules as small as 1 mm may be evident.[18]

Hyperplastic Nodules

The most common lesion in the thyroid is the hyperplastic nodule, also termed a colloid or adenomatous nodule. The etiology of thyroid glandular hyperplasia includes iodine deficiency and disorders of hormone synthesis. Production of the thyroid hormones T3 and T4 (thyroxine) by thyroid follicle epithelial cells is regulated by release of thyroid-stimulating hormone (TSH) from the anterior pituitary gland. Impaired or deficient thyroid hormone synthesis causes TSH levels to increase, and increases in TSH then produce follicular cell hypertrophy and hyperplasia. Repetitive cycles of hyperplasia followed by involution may produce irregular thyroid enlargement and multinodular goiter.[9] Otherwise identical-appearing follicular epithelial cells differ in their sensitivity to growth stimuli and in their intrinsic proliferative capabilities, which leads to nodule formation over time.[19] It was formerly believed that hyperplastic nodules could be distinguished from true neoplasms by virtue of their polyclonality. More recent studies, however, suggest that both neoplasms and hyperplastic nodules are monoclonal. Despite their prevalence, therefore, the pathophysiology of thyroid nodule formation remains poorly understood.

On sonography, hyperplastic nodules have a wide spectrum of appearances. They are most often isoechoic, but can also be hypoechoic and commonly undergo cystic and hemorrhagic degeneration (**Fig. 5**). Larger solid masses may be entirely echogenic. Cystic areas may contain either serous fluid or colloid; old hemorrhage and resultant echogenic fluid may also be noted. Punctuate highly echogenic foci with ring-down artifact represent colloid crystals within colloid cysts (**Fig. 6**). If residual strands of thyroid tissue remain within the cystic areas, a characteristic honeycomb appearance may result (**Fig. 7**).[20]

Box 1
Types of thyroid nodules

Benign nodules

    Colloid (hyperplastic, adenomatous) nodules

    Hashimoto (chronic lymphocytic) thyroiditis

    Cysts: colloid, simple, or hemorrhagic

    Follicular adenomas

    Hürthle-cell (oxyphil-cell) adenomas (variant of follicular adenoma)

Malignant nodules

    Papillary carcinoma

    Follicular carcinoma

    Medullary carcinoma

    Anaplastic carcinoma

    Primary thyroid lymphoma

    Metastatic carcinoma (breast, renal cell, others)

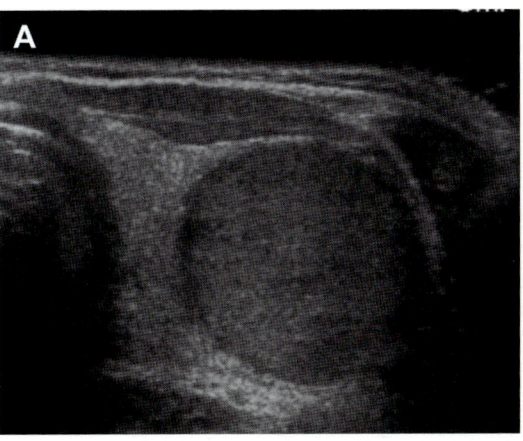 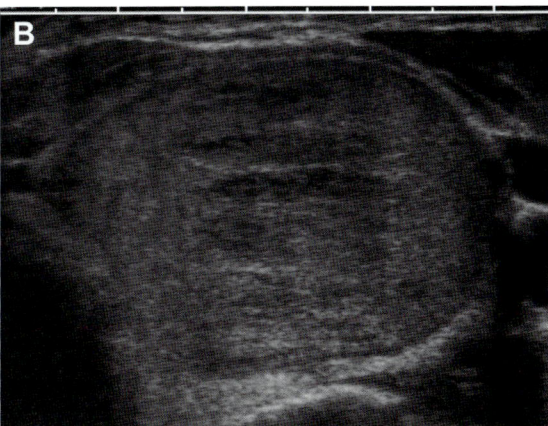

Fig. 5. Hyperplastic nodule. (A) Transverse image shows solid nodule in thyroid with hypoechoic halo, biopsy proven to represent a benign thyroid nodule. (B) Ultrasound 6 months later demonstrates internal cystic degeneration.

Nonuniform patterns of degeneration may produce mural nodules, septations, or internal debris. Degeneration of hyperplastic nodules may also produce dystrophic calcification and manifest as either coarse internal calcification or peripheral "eggshell" calcification (**Fig. 8**).[18] The term goiter is used when hyperplasia leads to overall increase in the size of the thyroid gland. Multinodular goiter, which is composed of multiple hyperplastic nodules with varying degrees of colloid, necrosis, or hemorrhage, is generally heterogeneous in appearance with multiple masses of varying size and echo texture.

Hashimoto Thyroiditis

Hashimoto thyroiditis is a common autoimmune disease in which patients, predominantly women, develop antibodies to thyroglobulin and the thyroid peroxidase enzyme. It causes a characteristic sonographic pattern of innumerable tiny hypoechoic nodules that may become confluent, interspersed with echogenic fibrous bands (**Fig. 9**). Vascularity may be increased, decreased, or normal, and FNA is usually not necessary for diagnosis.[20]

THYROID NEOPLASMS

Thyroid cancer is relatively uncommon in the United States. In 2007, an estimated 33,550 cases will be diagnosed, accounting for about 1530

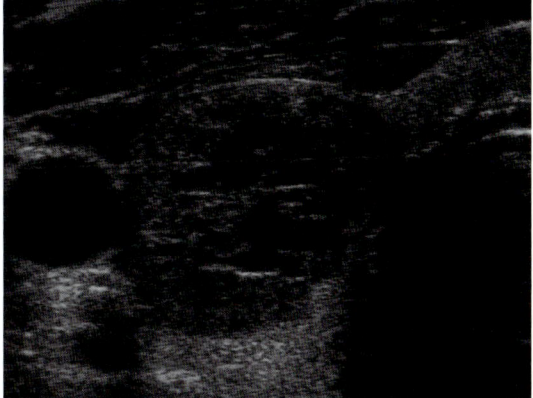

Fig. 6. Transverse image of right thyroid lobe shows cyst in lower pole of thyroid containing an echogenic focus with ring-down artifact posteriorly. This appearance is diagnostic of a colloid cyst.

Fig. 7. Transverse image of right thyroid lobe shows innumerable cystic spaces separated by a fine mesh of thin septations. This honeycomb appearance represents a benign thyroid nodule, which was proven by FNA.

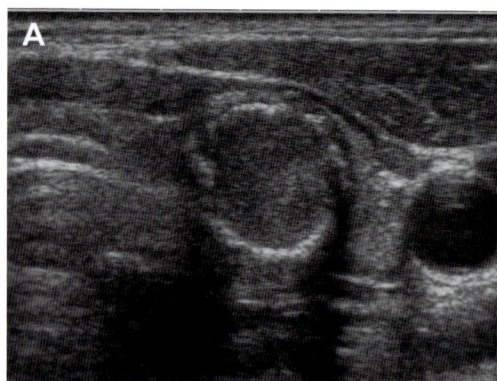
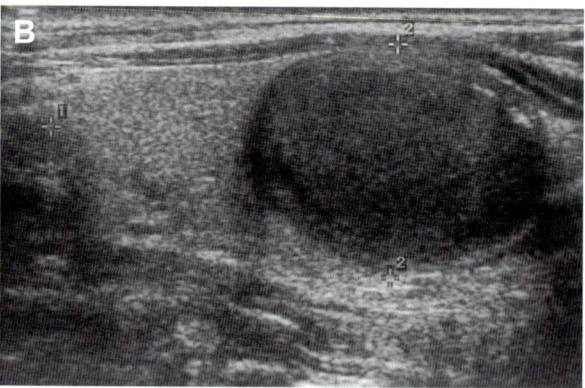

Fig. 8. Eggshell calcification. (A) Transverse image of left thyroid lobe shows complete thin rim of calcification encircling thyroid nodule. (B) Longitudinal image of benign thyroid nodule in a different patient shows incomplete delicate thin rim of calcification at inferior pole of nodule proven to represent a benign hemorrhagic cyst.

deaths. The incidence of thyroid cancer in the United States has increased from 3.6 per 100,000 in 1973 to 8.7 per 100,000 in 2002, but virtually all of this increase is believed to be attributable to increased detection of small papillary cancers on imaging studies.[21] Thyroid malignancies may arise from follicular epithelium (papillary, follicular, anaplastic) or from parafollicular C-cells (medullary carcinoma) and are classified as differentiated (papillary and follicular), medullary, and undifferentiated (anaplastic) carcinomas. The major risk factor for development of thyroid carcinoma is radiation exposure to the head and neck. Several oncogenes and tumor suppressor genes have been identified as playing a role in formation of both benign and malignant thyroid nodules.[22]

PAPILLARY CARCINOMA

Papillary cancer is the most common thyroid malignancy, accounting for 75% to 80% of thyroid cancers. Papillary cancers are typically slow-growing tumors with an excellent prognosis. In some autopsy studies, papillary cancers less than 10 mm in size, called papillary microcarcinomas, were found in 22% to 36% of patients who had no known thyroid pathology during life.[5,7] One study of patients who had papillary microcarcinoma found no statistically significant difference in mortality between patients who underwent surgical resection versus a cohort managed by observation alone.[6] Approximately 15% of thyroid carcinomas behave in an aggressive manner, however.[23] Risk factors for aggressive behavior of papillary microcarcinomas include extracapsular invasion, metastatic lymph node size, hoarseness, and postoperative thyroglobulin levels.[6]

Histologic features of papillary cancer include presence of psammoma bodies and characteristic nuclear changes, such as ground-glass appearance, longitudinal grooves, and inclusions.[24] The most specific sonographic finding of papillary cancer is the presence of punctuate, non-shadowing

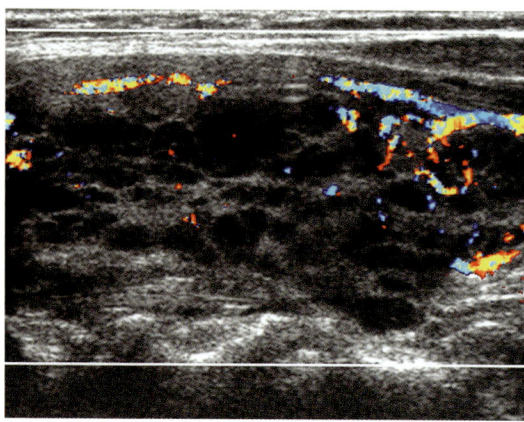

Fig. 9. Hashimoto thyroiditis. Longitudinal image shows innumerable small hypoechoic nodules set against background of echogenic thyroid parenchyma. Vascularity is slightly increased.

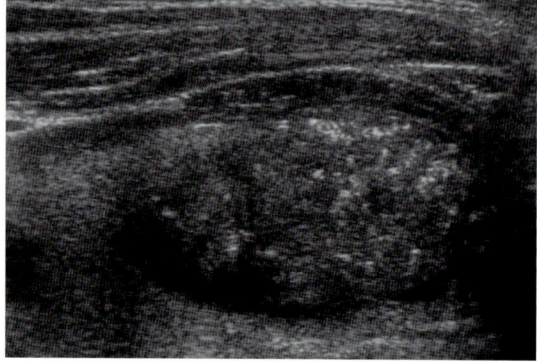

Fig. 10. Transverse image of right thyroid lobe in 39-year-old man who had papillary cancer. Innumerable microcalcifications create a "snowstorm" appearance.

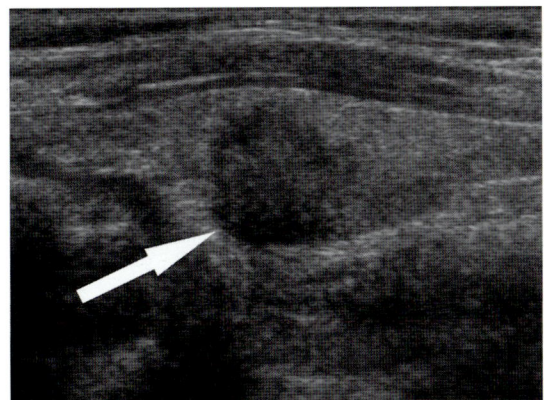

Fig. 11. Longitudinal image of hypoechoic papillary cancer (*arrow*) with irregular margins. The lesion is larger in anteroposterior dimension than in craniocaudal dimension (taller than wide).

echogenic foci termed microcalcifications, which are believed to represent dystrophic calcifications associated with psammoma bodies (**Fig. 10**). Although this finding has a high specificity (85%–95%)[1,25] sensitivity is only 25% to 59%.[1] Most papillary cancers are solid (87%) and hypoechoic (86%) compared with the surrounding thyroid parenchyma (**Fig. 11**).[26] Some evidence of intrinsic vascularity is generally seen, though the distribution of vascularity has not been found to be a reliable finding.[26–29] Papillary thyroid cancer metastasizes by way of lymphatics to cervical lymph nodes, which may contain microcalcifications, internal vascularity, and cystic change because of extensive degeneration (**Fig. 12**).

FOLLICULAR NEOPLASMS

Follicular adenomas are encapsulated true neoplasms of the thyroid gland and represent about 5% to 10% of all thyroid nodules. A minority of adenomas may be autonomously hyperfunctioning causing thyrotoxicosis, and thus the initial workup of a palpable thyroid nodule should include measurement of serum TSH levels.[2,3] Low TSH level would be an indication for thyroid scintigraphy, which is otherwise not useful in the evaluation of thyroid nodules. Differentiation of follicular adenoma from a follicular carcinoma is based on the presence of capsular or vascular invasion on histologic examination and thus cannot be made by sonography or by FNA cytology. Like thyroid nodules in general, follicular tumors are more common in women.

On sonography, follicular adenomas and follicular carcinomas are usually solitary encapsulated tumors, often with a well-defined peripheral hypoechoic halo representing the fibrous capsule (**Fig. 13**). Two histologic patterns of growth of follicular carcinomas can be observed. The minimally invasive type is encapsulated, in contrast to the widely invasive type, which extends beyond the tumor capsule into blood vessels and adjacent parenchyma. Echogenicity is variable and follicular neoplasms can be echogenic, isoechoic, or hypoechoic. Echogenic adenomas are often smoothly marginated and ovoid in appearance, prompting use of the term "pseudotesticle" to describe their appearance (**Fig. 14**). In contrast to papillary carcinomas, follicular carcinomas metastasize hematogenously to bone, lung, brain, and liver rather than by way of lymphatics. Hürthle (oncocytic) cells may constitute most or all of a follicular tumor, in which case the tumor is classified as a Hürthle cell carcinoma, a variant of follicular carcinoma.[30] Another histologic variant is insular thyroid cancer, which is poorly differentiated and associated with an aggressive clinical course.[24]

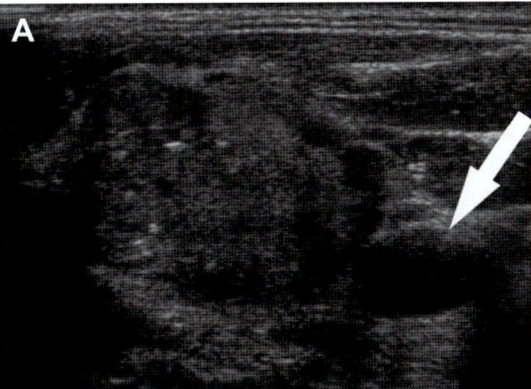 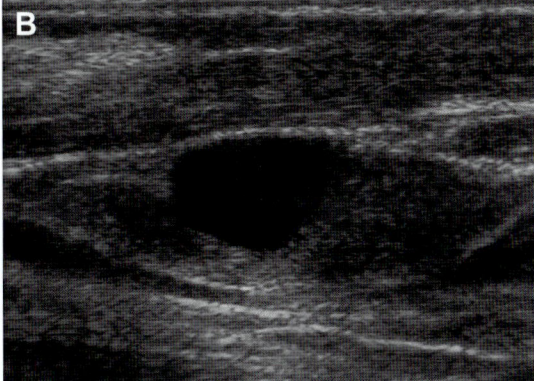

Fig. 12. Metastatic papillary carcinoma involving cervical lymph nodes. (*A*) Transverse gray-scale image of papillary cancer metastatic to a right lateral cervical lymph node containing microcalcifications. The large node is just lateral to the right carotid artery (*arrow*). (*B*) Longitudinal image of metastatic papillary carcinoma with cystic change in cervical lymph node.

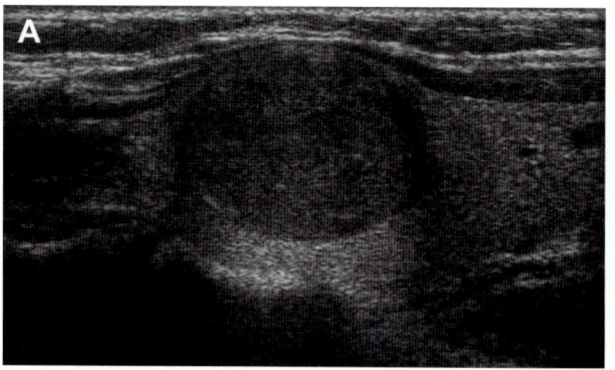
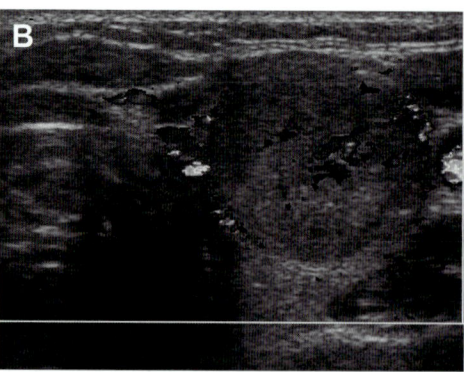

Fig. 13. Follicular adenoma. (*A*) Longitudinal gray-scale image shows well-defined hypoechoic nodule with incomplete halo. (*B*) Transverse image shows flow in peripheral hypoechoic capsule and internally.

MEDULLARY CARCINOMA

Medullary thyroid cancer is a neuroendocrine tumor arising from the parafollicular C cells located in the upper two thirds of the thyroid gland.[31] Although medullary cancer is associated with MEN2A (C-cell hyperplasia, pheochromocytoma, hyperparathyroidism), 80% occur sporadically. Ninety-five percent of patients who have MEN2A have C-cell hyperplasia and in 80% of affected patients, medullary thyroid carcinoma is the initial manifestation. Patients who have sporadic medullary carcinoma typically present with a painless palpable nodule in the fifth or sixth decade of life, but the disease is often metastatic to cervical lymph nodes at presentation.[32] There is a slight female preponderance (1.5:1).[31] The value of serum calcitonin screening measurement in patients who have thyroid nodules is dubious because levels are often falsely elevated and FNA is highly accurate; however, calcitonin levels are useful once the diagnosis of medullary thyroid cancer has been established by cytologic evaluation.[32] On sonography, medullary carcinomas are typically solid, hypoechoic, and often have coarse central calcifications (**Fig. 15**).

ANAPLASTIC CARCINOMA

Anaplastic carcinoma of the thyroid is a rare tumor of the thyroid, but extremely aggressive, representing the terminal stage in the dedifferentiation of a follicular or papillary carcinoma. Patients are usually elderly with a history of goiter and present with a rapidly growing neck mass. The tumor characteristically invades locally and involves adjacent muscles and blood vessels. Distant metastases most commonly involve the lungs, bones, brain, and liver.[30]

On sonography, anaplastic carcinomas are generally large, at least 5 to 10 cm, fixed, hard, and heterogeneous in appearance (**Fig. 16**). Internal

Fig. 14. Longitudinal image of follicular neoplasm (Hürthle cell) with pseudotesticle appearance.

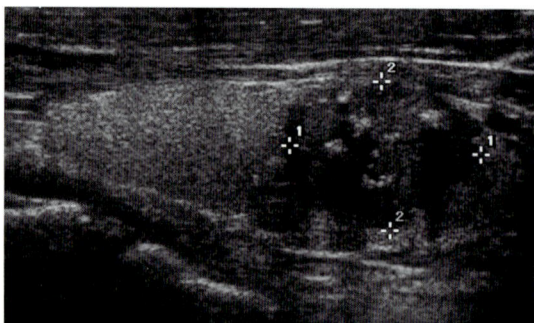

Fig. 15. Medullary carcinoma. Longitudinal image shows hypoechoic nodule at inferior pole of thyroid with coarse central calcifications. (*Courtesy of* Lucy E. Hann, MD, New York, NY.)

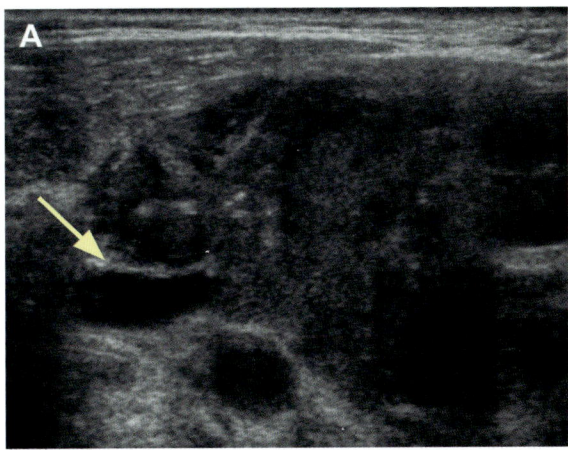 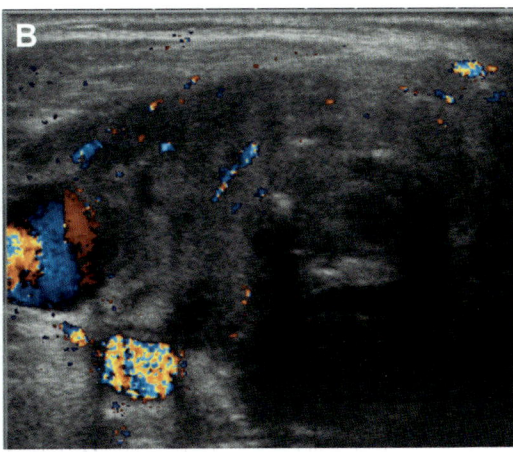

Fig. 16. Anaplastic thyroid cancer in 74-year-old woman. (A) Transverse gray-scale image of an enlarged, irregular, heterogeneous thyroid mass with mass effect on the internal jugular vein (arrow). Carotid artery is posterior and medial. (B) Color Doppler image of the thyroid near the same level. At this level, internal coarse calcifications with shadowing are seen.

calcifications and cystic or necrotic areas may be seen. Adjacent enlarged lymph nodes are common. Invasion of adjacent structures, such as the carotid sheath, trachea, and muscles, and the overall extent of tumor are often better assessed on CT or MR imaging.

LYMPHOMA

Primary lymphoma of the thyroid is uncommon, accounting for 2% of extranodal lymphomas and less than 5% of all malignant thyroid tumors. Most thyroid lymphomas are non-Hodgkin lymphomas. Patients present with a rapidly enlarging painless neck mass. Lymphomas may occur in the setting of Hashimoto thyroiditis. On ultrasound, thyroid lymphoma is characteristically very hypoechoic with a pseudocystic pattern (increased through transmission) similar to lymphoma seen in other organs, such as the liver or lymph nodes (Fig. 17).[30]

THYROID METASTASIS

Metastatic disease to the thyroid is rare. In a large study of 18,105 thyroidectomies in two Italian pathology databases, only 24 cases (0.13%) were found to represent metastatic disease to the thyroid with the main sites of origin being lung, esophagus, breast, and kidney.[33] On sonography, metastases to the thyroid have a nonspecific appearance and are usually solid, noncalcified, hypoechoic nodules (Fig. 18). With increased use of whole-body fluorodeoxyglucose positron emission tomography (FDG-PET) and PET-CT in patients who have a known primary malignancy, focal areas of hypermetabolism in the thyroid have been identified with increasing frequency,

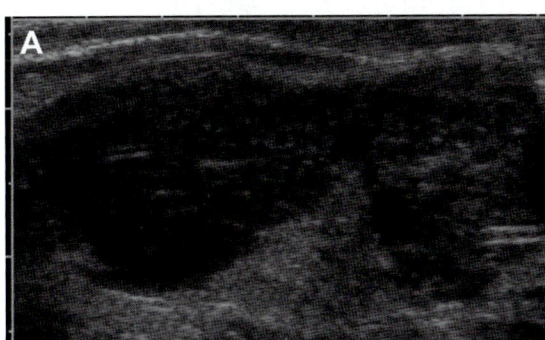 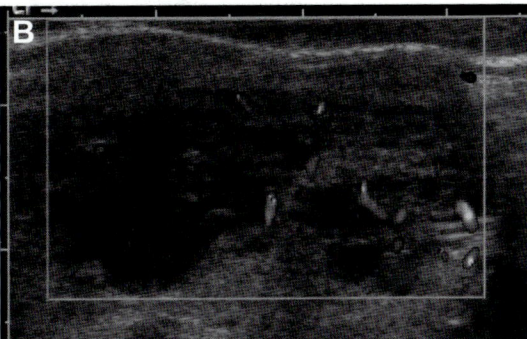

Fig. 17. Thyroid lymphoma. (A) Gray-scale image of a bulky, hypoechoic mass with pseudocystic appearance. (B) Color Doppler image demonstrates internal vascularity.

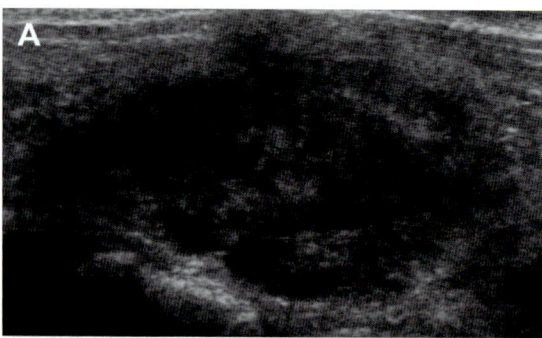 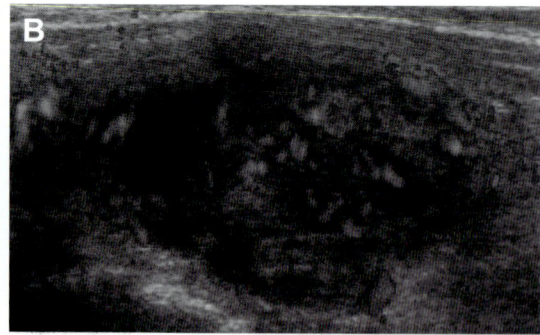

Fig. 18. Thyroid metastasis. (A) Gray-scale image of a heterogeneously hypoechoic mass in thyroid, biopsy proven to represent metastases from lung cancer primary. (B) Power Doppler demonstrates marked internal vascularity. (Case courtesy of R. Brooke Jeffrey MD.)

with prevalence ranging from 2.2% to 4.3%. In several studies, the rate of malignancy in these metabolically active thyroid "incidentalomas" ranges from 26.7% to 80%, with the vast majority of malignancies representing primary thyroid carcinomas, not metastatic disease. Although the standardized uptake values were higher in malignant nodules than benign nodules in most studies, FNA is usually indicated for definitive assessment.[34–40]

The sonographic characteristics of these specific types of thyroid nodules are summarized in **Table 1**.

SONOGRAPHIC FEATURES OF THYROID NODULES

Current management guidelines recommend sonography and FNA for management of thyroid nodules, because no single noninvasive test can reliably distinguish benign from malignant nodules. But with the odds of malignancy only approximately 1 in 20, and thyroid cancer accounting for only 0.5% of all cancer deaths, a sensible strategy for determining which nodules should undergo FNA is essential. Numerous sonographic features of thyroid nodules have been described and studied as a means of triaging nodules for FNA. These include size, multiplicity, echogenicity, presence of calcifications, margins, contour, shape, internal architecture, and vascularity. The most common appearance for papillary thyroid carcinoma is a solitary, solid hypoechoic nodule with ill-defined borders, microcalcifications, and internal vascularity. In one series of 55 papillary carcinomas, however, more than half had at least one feature not commonly associated with malignancy.[26] Conversely, in a series of 68 benign nodules, 69% of them had at least one finding usually associated with malignancy.[41] Although no single feature can distinguish benign from malignant nodules, taking all sonographic features into account can shed some light on which nodules should undergo further testing.

Size and Multiplicity

Thyroid nodules become palpable when they reach approximately 1 cm in size. When palpation was the sole means of identifying nodules, this diameter was the de facto threshold for biopsy. Although the American Association of Clinical Endocrinologists and American Thyroid Association guidelines continue to use 1 to 1.5 cm as a practical threshold for selecting nodules for FNA,[2,3] it has been shown that size is not a good predictor of malignancy. Papini and colleagues[42] evaluated the risk for malignancy in 195 solitary nonpalpable thyroid nodules 8 to 15 mm in size and 207 multinodular goiters, and found that the cancer prevalence was similar in nodules greater or smaller than 10 mm. Rather than a simple size threshold, their study found that a strategy of performing FNA in all hypoechoic solid nodules with irregular margins, intranodular flow, or microcalcifications would lead to biopsy in only 31% of nodules while still detecting 87% of the cancers. In nodules larger than 1 cm, Frates and colleagues[43] found no significant difference in the rate of malignancy in 1039 solid nodules by size, although there was a trend toward higher rate of malignancy in nodules larger than 3 cm. The recent Society of Radiologists in Ultrasound consensus statement suggests that, rather than a fixed size threshold, sonographic features should be used to guide nodule selection for FNA. More suspicious sonographic features (see later discussion) should trigger biopsy at small nodule size, whereas nearly completely cystic nodules without other suspicious features probably do not require biopsy at any size.[1]

The presence of multiple nodules does not make thyroid carcinoma less likely, contrary to former teaching.[44] In multinodular glands, each nodule should be scrutinized for suspicious features and

Table 1
Summary of sonographic features of thyroid nodules

	Echogenicity	Rim	Vascularity	Calcifications	Cyst Component	Special Distinguishing Findings
Papillary cancer	Usually hypoechoic	Ill defined more worrisome; can be well defined	Usually hypervascular compared with rest of thyroid; pattern not reliable indicator	May see coarse calcifications or microcalcifications	Usually less than 50%	Microcalcifications
Follicular cancer	Usually hypoechoic	Well defined	—	—	No	Pseudotesticle
Medullary cancer	—	—	—	Central coarse calcification	—	May see central coarse calcification
Anaplastic cancer	Heterogeneous	Ill defined	Internal vascularity	Various types	May see internal necrotic change	Invasion of adjacent structures
Lymphoma	Hypoechoic	—	Hypovascular	No	May see cystic necrosis	Increased through transmission
Degenerating adenoma: hemorrhagic degeneration	Variable	Well defined	Yes	May see thin rim eggshell calcification	May be present	Colloid crystals (echogenic foci with ring down)
Cystic degeneration	Variable	Well defined	Variable	—	>75% cystic	—

selected for FNA on the basis of sonographic features, rather than size alone.

Growth

Interval follow-up is usually recommended for sonographically detected nodules, yet there are no data to suggest which growth rates or patterns are suspicious. Both benign and malignant nodules can increase or decrease in size. Brander and colleagues[45] conducted a 5-year follow-up study of 69 patients who had thyroid abnormalities found incidentally as part of an ultrasound screening study of 253 randomly selected adults. Of the original cohort of 69 patients who had abnormalities, 57 patients participated in the follow-up study. The investigators found that, regardless of echo texture, 35% of the 34 cytologically benign nodules had increased in size at follow-up and remained benign at repeat FNA. Eight (24%) had decreased in size or disappeared altogether. New lesions were detected in 7 subjects, and cytology proved to be benign in the 5 who underwent FNA. The remaining 2 lesions were too small and the patients preferred follow-up. Overall, their results found no malignancies at 5-year follow-up, even among those whose nodules had increased in size. A more recent study of the natural history of 330 benign solid and cystic thyroid nodules showed that 89% of the solid benign thyroid nodules increased in volume by 15% or greater over a 5-year period.[46] Solid nodules were more likely to grow than cystic nodules. At the time of a 9- to 12-month follow-up scan, 39% of benign nodules had increased in volume by 15% or more. Within a higher risk subset of 74 larger nodules with more rapid growth, only one proved to be malignant at re-biopsy.

Calcifications

Calcifications have been found in papillary, medullary, and anaplastic thyroid carcinomas as either psammoma bodies or as amorphous granular deposits. Of all the sonographic features associated with thyroid malignancy, microcalcifications are the most specific. Microcalcifications are defined as punctuate echogenic foci without acoustic shadowing or associated comet-tail artifact. The positive predictive value of a finding of microcalcifications in a thyroid nodule ranges from 24.3% to 70%.[1] Other types of calcification may also be present. In one series, microcalcifications were seen in 42% of papillary thyroid cancers, coarse calcifications in 9.1%, and peripheral calcifications in 1.8% (**Fig. 19**).[26] Although formerly considered a benign finding, eggshell calcifications have been reported in thyroid cancers.[47] Coarse central

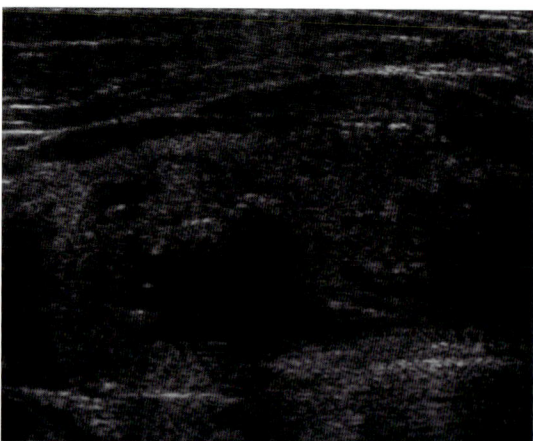

Fig. 19. Longitudinal image of a papillary cancer with coarse, shadowing calcifications. (*Case courtesy of R. Brooke Jeffrey, MD.*)

calcifications are a common feature of medullary carcinoma, although this entity represents only 1 of 250 thyroid nodules.[48]

Echogenicity

Most thyroid carcinomas are hypoechoic relative to surrounding thyroid parenchyma. In a series of 55 papillary carcinomas studied by Chan and colleagues,[26] 86% of papillary cancers were hypoechoic. A more recent series of 68 papillary cancers from the same institution found that 78% were hypoechoic, with 12% isoechoic, 9% mixed echogenicity, and 1% hyperechoic.[49] Hypoechogenicity is a sensitive sign but is nonspecific: 30.6% to 55% of benign nodules are also hypoechoic.[25,41] An echogenic appearance is commonly associated with follicular neoplasms, both benign and malignant, but can also be seen in papillary cancers. Kim and colleagues[50] suggested that "marked hypoechogenicity," defined as echogenicity less than that of adjacent musculature, is a more specific appearance for thyroid carcinoma, but others found that this feature had only fair interobserver agreement.

Cystic Change and Ring-Down Artifact

Thyroid cancer is not common in predominantly cystic nodules. In a series of 209 nodules assessed by Frates and colleagues,[27] only 2 of 32 malignant nodules were greater than 50% cystic, as compared with 30 of 177 benign nodules. Nodules that are nearly completely cystic are virtually never cancers in the absence of other concerning features.[1,26] Nevertheless, a cystic component may be seen in 13% to 26% of thyroid cancers.[1,26,51] When FNA is to be performed on a cystic nodule, the biopsy should be targeted to the solid components. Additional features are helpful in assessing cystic nodules. In their series of papillary carcinomas, Chan and colleagues[26] found no cystic carcinomas without internal flow in their solid components. The Mayo Clinic group has observed that a "honeycomb" appearance of multiple cystic spaces bordered by numerous thin septations virtually always correlates with benign cytology on FNA.[20] Punctate echogenic foci associated with comet-tail artifact representing inspissated colloid seems to be present only in benign cystic nodules. Ahuja and colleagues[52] reviewed the histologies of 100 cystic nodules containing comet-tail artifact, and found they all represented benign hyperplastic (colloid) nodules. During the same time period, they found 70 malignancies on sonography and FNA, none of which were associated with the artifact (**Fig. 20**).

Vascularity

Almost all solid nodules display some flow on color Doppler interrogation with current generation ultrasound equipment. Initial optimism that color Doppler flow patterns could differentiate benign from malignant nodules quickly faded as larger studies were performed. In general, a peripheral flow pattern tends to be a feature of benign nodules, and malignant nodules tend to have internal vascularity (**Fig. 21**), but there is considerable overlap. Among 254 nodules biopsied by Frates and colleagues,[27] a pattern of marked internal vascularity was seen in 14 of 32 malignant nodules (42%) but also in 26 of 177 benign ones (14.7%). Although marked internal vascularity was more

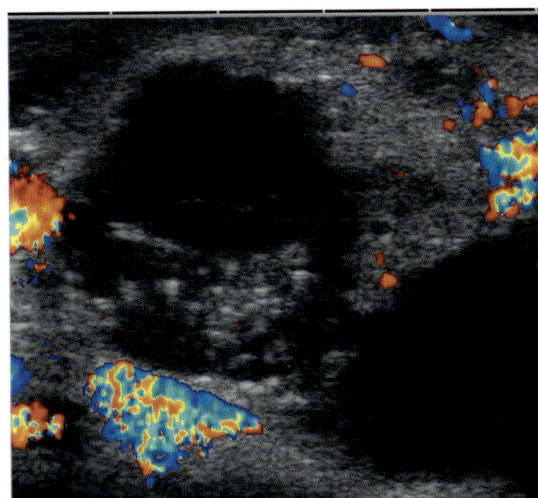

Fig. 20. Transverse image of benign cystic nodule with dependent internal colloid as evidenced by comet-tail artifacts.

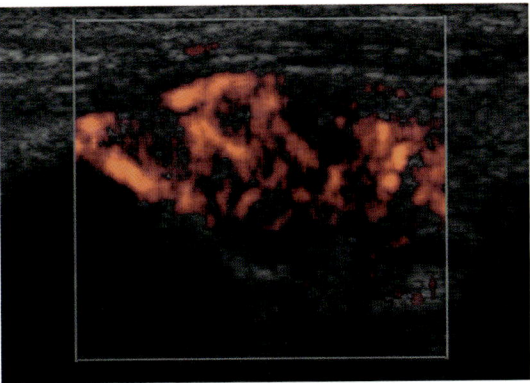

Fig. 21. Power Doppler image of chaotic internal vasculature in a papillary carcinoma.

often present in malignant than benign nodules, more than half of nodules with internal hypervascularity were benign. Furthermore, 14% of their solid hypovascular nodules were malignant. Another series of 68 papillary thyroid cancers found that 19% were hypovascular.[4] In the study by Chan and colleagues,[26] 9.1% of 55 papillary cancers were hypovascular, but none were entirely avascular. A cystic nodule without any internal flow therefore is unlikely to be a papillary carcinoma.

Shape and Margins

By analogy with breast carcinomas, Kim and colleagues[50] studied the shape of thyroid carcinomas and found that a shape taller than wide was 92.5% specific for malignancy (see **Fig. 11**). This feature had fairly low (32.7%) sensitivity, however, and was not definitively confirmed in a series by Iannuccilli and colleagues[25] The latter found only 2 "tall" nodules on retrospective review of 70 thyroid nodules (34 malignant and 36 benign), and both were benign. Spherical shape was also found to be predictive of malignancy in a study of 993 thyroid nodules that had undergone FNA. The overall rate of thyroid malignancy in their series was 11%, but the incidence in the most spherical nodules was 18% versus only 5% in the least spherical. In the same study, a ratio of long axis to short axis length of greater than 2.5 was 100% predictive of benignity, although this shape was relatively rare.[53]

A sonolucent halo, previously believed to be a feature of benign nodules, can be seen in 10% to 24% of papillary cancers (**Fig. 22**).[25,26,51] The finding of an irregular margin has widely varying sensitivity for malignancy (7% to 97%)[1,26,50,54] and the highest interobserver variability of several sonographic features (see **Fig. 11**).[41]

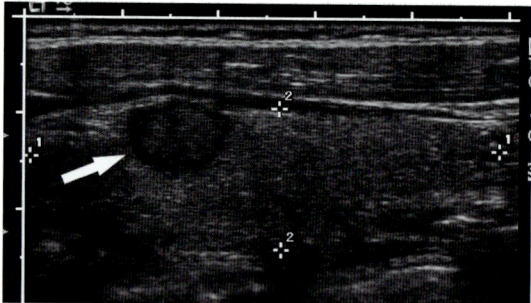

Fig. 22. Longitudinal image of small upper pole papillary carcinoma (*arrow*) with hypoechoic halo.

Local Invasion and Lymphadenopathy

Extension of a mass beyond the thyroid capsule into adjacent trachea or muscle is highly suggestive of an aggressive malignancy (see **Fig. 12**). Likewise, the presence of local lymphadenopathy with any suspicious features, such as rounded shape, loss of fatty hilum, cystic change, microcalcifications, or irregular internal hypervascularity, should prompt FNA of the node and any associated thyroid nodules.[3]

Multivariate Analyses

Clearly no single sonographic feature predicts malignancy, but some features are better than others. Microcalcifications are more commonly associated with papillary cancer than with benign disease and should trigger biopsy at relatively small nodule size. Several groups have tried to develop multivariate predictors of malignancy. Kim and colleagues[50] studied four predictors of malignancy in solid nodules—microcalcifications, irregular margins, hypoechogenicity, and shape more tall than wide—and performed FNA if any of these features were present. In their hands, this system yielded 93.8% sensitivity and 66% specificity with a positive predictive value of 56.1%. But in a follow-up study of 68 benign and 2 malignant nodules assessed using the same method, Wienke found that 69% of benign nodules had at least one finding associated with malignancy.[41] Finally, Koike and colleagues[54] devised a regression formula to predict malignancy using five sonographic features as variables—margin, shape, internal architecture, echogenicity, and calcification—and used it to predict malignancy in follicular and nonfollicular neoplasms. Using the model, the sensitivity of ultrasound was 86.5% for nonfollicular neoplasms, with specificity of 92.3%. Selecting a probability of malignancy of 0.2 with the regression formula yielded sensitivity of 94% and specificity of 87%. They found that follicular neoplasms were not reliably assessed with their formula, however.

SELECTION CRITERIA FOR FINE NEEDLE ASPIRATION OF THYROID NODULES

Given the relative lack of specificity of many ultrasound findings of thyroid malignancy, it can be difficult to determine which nodules should undergo FNA. Guidelines for the selection of nodules for FNA is the subject of a separate article in this issue. Briefly, the recent consensus conference statement of the Society of Radiologists in Ultrasound provides recommendations for management of thyroid nodules 1 cm or larger in maximum diameter (**Table 2**), which are based

Table 2
Management recommendations for thyroid nodules 1 cm or larger in maximal diameter[1]

Sonographic Feature	Recommendation
Solitary nodule	
Microcalcifications	Strongly consider US-guided FNA if ≥1 cm
Solid or coarse calcification	Strongly consider US-guided FNA if ≥1.5 cm
Mixed cystic and solid or almost entirely cystic with solid mural component	Consider US-guided FNA if ≥2 cm
None of the above but substantial growth since prior US	Consider US-guided FNA
Almost completely cystic and without significant growth or features above	US-guided FNA probably not necessary
Multiple nodules	Consider US-guided FNA of one or more nodules, prioritizing selection based on criteria for solid nodules in order listed above

Abbreviation: US, ultrasound.

on the predictive value of different sonographic features, with microcalcifications being most suspicious and a predominantly cystic appearance having least likelihood of malignancy.

SUMMARY

Thyroid nodules can be identified by ultrasound in almost half the adult population of the United States. Approximately 95% of these are benign, and most malignancies are indolent if not altogether clinically occult. Nevertheless, some malignant lesions can be associated with an aggressive course. Risk factors for malignancy include age younger than 20 or greater than 60 years, history of neck irradiation, and family history of thyroid cancer. No single ultrasound feature can distinguish benign from malignant nodules, but the presence of microcalcifications should prompt FNA at smaller nodule sizes than other features. FDG-avid thyroid nodules detected on PET scans performed for cancer staging in patients who have other primary malignancies have a high rate of malignancy and are more likely to represent thyroid carcinomas than metastatic disease. The presence of multiple nodules does not decrease the likelihood of malignancy, and the features of each nodule should be scrutinized to determine which nodules should undergo biopsy.

REFERENCES

1. Frates MC, Benson CB, Charboneau JW, et al. Management of thyroid nodules detected at US: society of radiologists in ultrasound consensus conference statement. Radiology 2005;237:794–800.
2. Cooper DS, Doherty GM, Haugen BR, et al. Management guidelines for patients with thyroid nodules and differentiated thyroid cancer. Thyroid 2006;16:109–42.
3. Gharib H, Papini E, Baskin H, et al. American Association of Clinical Endocrinologists and Associazione Medici Endocrinologi medical guidelines for clinical practice for the diagnosis and management of thyroid nodules. Endocr Pract 2006;12:63–78.
4. Bramley MD, Harrison BJ. Papillary microcarcinoma of the thyroid gland. Br J Surg 1996;83:1674–83.
5. Harach HR, Franssila KO, Wasenius VM. Occult papillary carcinoma of the thyroid. A "normal" finding in Finland. A systematic autopsy study. Cancer 1985;56:531–8.
6. Ito Y, Uruno T, Nakano K, et al. An observation trial without surgical treatment in patients with papillary microcarcinoma of the thyroid. Thyroid 2003;13:381–7.
7. Martinez-Tello FJ, Martinez-Cabruja R, Fernandez-Martin J, et al. Occult carcinoma of the thyroid. A systematic autopsy study from Spain of two series performed with two different methods. Cancer 1993;71:4022–9.
8. Ross DS. Nonpalpable thyroid nodules—managing an epidemic. J Clin Endocrinol Metab 2002;87:1938–40.
9. Maitra A, Abbas A. The endocrine system. In: Kumar V, Fausto N, Abbas A, editors. Robbins & Cotran pathologic basis of disease. 7th edition. Philadelphia: Elsevier Saunders; 2004. p. 1155–226.
10. Lyshchik A, Drozd V, Schloegl S, et al. Three-dimensional ultrasonography for volume measurement of thyroid nodules in children. J Ultrasound Med 2004;23:247–54.
11. Hagel J, Bicknell SG. Impact of 3D sonography on workroom time efficiency. AJR Am J Roentgenol 2007;188:966–9.
12. Dahl JJ, Guenther DA, Trahey GE. Adaptive imaging and spatial compounding in the presence of aberration. IEEE Trans Ultrason Ferroelectr Freq Control 2005;52:1131–44.
13. Szopinski KT, Wysocki M, Pajk AM, et al. Tissue harmonic imaging of thyroid nodules: initial experience. J Ultrasound Med 2003;22:5–12.
14. Lyshchik A, Higashi T, Asato R, et al. Thyroid gland tumor diagnosis at US elastography. Radiology 2005;237:202–11.
15. Rago T, Santini F, Scutari M, et al. Elastography: new developments in ultrasound for predicting malignancy in thyroid nodules. J Clin Endocrinol Metab 2007;92(8):2917–22.
16. Bae U, Dighe M, Dubinsky T, et al. Ultrasound thyroid elastography using carotid artery pulsation: preliminary study. J Ultrasound Med 2007;26:797–805.
17. Tan GH, Gharib H. Thyroid incidentalomas: management approaches to nonpalpable nodules discovered incidentally on thyroid imaging. Ann Intern Med 1997;126:226–31.
18. Tessler FN, Tublin ME. Thyroid sonography: current applications and future directions. AJR Am J Roentgenol 1999;173:437–43.
19. Hegedus L, Gerber H, Bonnema SJ. Multinodular goiter. In: Degroot L, Jameson LJ, editors. Endocrinology. Philadelphia: Saunders; 2005. p. 2113–27.
20. Reading CC, Charboneau JW, Hay ID, et al. Sonography of thyroid nodules: a "classic pattern" diagnostic approach. Ultrasound Q 2005;21:157–65.
21. Davies L, Welch HG. Increasing incidence of thyroid cancer in the United States, 1973–2002. JAMA 2006;295:2164–7.
22. Malchoff CD. Oncogenes and tumor suppressor genes in thyroid nodules and nonmedullary thyroid cancer. Available at: http://www.uptodate.com. Accessed October 6, 2007.
23. Ross DS. Overview of thyroid nodule formation. Available at: www.uptodate.com. Accessed October 6, 2007.

24. Lee SL, Ananthakrishnan S. Overview of follicular thyroid cancer. Available at: http://www.uptodate.com. Accessed October 6, 2007.
25. Iannuccilli JD, Cronan JJ, Monchik JM. Risk for malignancy of thyroid nodules as assessed by sonographic criteria: the need for biopsy. J Ultrasound Med 2004;23:1455–64.
26. Chan BK, Desser TS, McDougall IR, et al. Common and uncommon sonographic features of papillary thyroid carcinoma. J Ultrasound Med 2003;22:1083–90.
27. Frates MC, Benson CB, Doubilet PM, et al. Can color Doppler sonography aid in the prediction of malignancy of thyroid nodules? J Ultrasound Med 2003;22:127–31 quiz 132–4.
28. Rago T, Vitti P, Chiovato L, et al. Role of conventional ultrasonography and color flow-Doppler sonography in predicting malignancy in "cold" thyroid nodules. Eur J Endocrinol 1998;138:41–6.
29. Shimamoto K, Endo T, Ishigaki T, et al. Thyroid nodules: evaluation with color Doppler ultrasonography. J Ultrasound Med 1993;12:673–8.
30. Schlumberger M, Caillou B. Miscellaneous tumors of the thyroid. In: Braverman LE, Utiger RD, editors. Werner and Ingbar's the thyroid: a fundamental and clinical text. 7th edition. Philadelphia: Lippincott-Raven; 1996. p. 961–5.
31. Ball DW, Baylin SB, de Bustros AC. Medullary thyroid carcinoma. In: Braverman LE, Utiger RD, editors. Werner and Ingbar's the thyroid: a fundamental and clinical text. 7th edition. Philadelphia: Lippincott-Raven; 1996. p. 946–60.
32. Sherman SI. Clinical manifestations and staging of medullary thyroid carcinoma. Available at: http://www.uptodate.com. Accessed October 6, 2007.
33. Papi G, Fadda G, Corsello SM, et al. Metastases to the thyroid gland: prevalence, clinicopathological aspects and prognosis: a 10-year experience. Clin Endocrinol (Oxf) 2007;66:565–71.
34. Bogsrud TV, Karantanis D, Nathan MA, et al. The value of quantifying 18F-FDG uptake in thyroid nodules found incidentally on whole-body PET-CT. Nucl Med Commun 2007;28:373–81.
35. Van den Bruel A, Maes A, De Potter T, et al. Clinical relevance of thyroid fluorodeoxyglucose-whole body positron emission tomography incidentaloma. J Clin Endocrinol Metab 2002;87:1517–20.
36. Are C, Hsu JF, Schoder H, et al. FDG-PET detected thyroid incidentalomas: need for further investigation? Ann Surg Oncol 2007;14:239–47.
37. Choi JY, Lee KS, Kim HJ, et al. Focal thyroid lesions incidentally identified by integrated 18F-FDG PET/CT: clinical significance and improved characterization. J Nucl Med 2006;47:609–15.
38. Cohen MS, Arslan N, Dehdashti F, et al. Risk of malignancy in thyroid incidentalomas identified by fluorodeoxyglucose-positron emission tomography. Surgery 2001;130:941–6.
39. Kang KW, Kim SK, Kang HS, et al. Prevalence and risk of cancer of focal thyroid incidentaloma identified by 18F-fluorodeoxyglucose positron emission tomography for metastasis evaluation and cancer screening in healthy subjects. J Clin Endocrinol Metab 2003;88:4100–4.
40. Yi JG, Marom EM, Munden RF, et al. Focal uptake of fluorodeoxyglucose by the thyroid in patients undergoing initial disease staging with combined PET/CT for non-small cell lung cancer. Radiology 2005;236:271–5.
41. Wienke JR, Chong WK, Fielding JR, et al. Sonographic features of benign thyroid nodules: interobserver reliability and overlap with malignancy. J Ultrasound Med 2003;22:1027–31.
42. Papini E, Guglielmi R, Bianchini A, et al. Risk of malignancy in nonpalpable thyroid nodules: predictive value of ultrasound and color-Doppler features. J Clin Endocrinol Metab 2002;87:1941–6.
43. Frates MC, Benson CB, Doubilet PM, et al. Likelihood of thyroid cancer based on sonographic assessment of nodule size and composition. Presented at the Radiological society of North America scientific assembly and annual meeting program. Chicago, November 28–December 3, 2004.
44. Utiger RD. The multiplicity of thyroid nodules and carcinomas. N Engl J Med 2005;352:2376–8.
45. Brander AE, Viikinkoski VP, Nickels JI, et al. Importance of thyroid abnormalities detected at US screening: a 5-year follow-up. Radiology 2000;215:801–6.
46. Alexander EK, Hurwitz S, Heering JP, et al. Natural history of benign solid and cystic thyroid nodules. Ann Intern Med 2003;138:315–8.
47. Cheng SP, Lee JJ, Lin J, et al. Eggshell calcification in follicular thyroid carcinoma. Eur Radiol 2005;15:1773–4.
48. Hegedus L. Clinical practice. The thyroid nodule. N Engl J Med 2004;351:1764–71.
49. Jun P, Chow LC, Jeffrey RB. The sonographic features of papillary thyroid carcinomas: pictorial essay. Ultrasound Q 2005;21:39–45.
50. Kim EK, Park CS, Chung WY, et al. New sonographic criteria for recommending fine-needle aspiration biopsy of nonpalpable solid nodules of the thyroid. AJR Am J Roentgenol 2002;178:687–91.
51. Watters DA, Ahuja AT, Evans RM, et al. Role of ultrasound in the management of thyroid nodules. Am J Surg 1992;164:654–7.
52. Ahuja A, Chick W, King W, et al. Clinical significance of the comet-tail artifact in thyroid ultrasound. J Clin Ultrasound 1996;24:129–33.
53. Alexander EK, Marqusee E, Orcutt J, et al. Thyroid nodule shape and prediction of malignancy. Thyroid 2004;14:953–8.
54. Koike E, Noguchi S, Yamashita H, et al. Ultrasonographic characteristics of thyroid nodules: prediction of malignancy. Arch Surg 2001;136:334–7.

Sonographic Imaging of Cervical Lymph Nodes in Patients with Thyroid Cancer

Jill E. Langer, MD[a,*], Susan J. Mandel, MD, MPH[b]

KEYWORDS

- Ultrasound • Thyroid cancer • Lymph nodes

Sonographic evaluation of the neck plays an important role in the evaluation of patients who have thyroid carcinoma at the time of initial diagnosis and in the assessment of recurrent disease. Most patients diagnosed with differentiated thyroid cancer have lesions that are confined to the thyroid or are minimally invasive into the adjacent soft tissues of the neck, yet often these cancers have already metastasized to the regional cervical nodes.[1,2] Sonography has been established as the most sensitive imaging test to diagnose these nodal metastases.[3–7] Detection of metastatic cervical lymph nodes by sonography at the time of initial presentation may alter the surgical approach to include a modified lateral neck dissection at the time of thyroidectomy.[4,8–10] Ultrasonography of the neck also offers an inexpensive and readily available means to detect recurrent thyroid cancer following thyroidectomy. Furthermore, when abnormalities are identified by neck sonography, they can be biopsied under direct sonographic visualization.[3,11]

ANATOMY

It is helpful for the imager evaluating the patient for metastatic thyroid cancer to have familiarity with the nomenclature used to describe the location of cervical nodes. The classic description of nodal location based on superficial anatomic landmarks has been replaced by imaging-based classifications.[12,13] The cervical lymph node classification most widely used by clinicians who specialize in head and neck cancer is that established by The American Joint Committee on Cancer Staging and the American Academy of Otolaryngology–Head and Neck Surgery, which groups the cervical nodes by regions (levels) to more closely reflect the clinical staging of head and neck tumors. Level I refers to nodes in the submental and submandibular regions. Levels II, III, and IV refer to nodes along the anterior cervical and internal jugular chains. Level II encompasses those nodes from the base of the skull to the lower border of the hyoid bone, Level III from the hyoid to the lower margin of the cricoid cartilage, and level IV from the cricoid to the clavicle. Level V nodes are those in the posterior compartment of the neck, along the course of the spinal accessory nerve, and are divided into upper (VA) and lower (VB) levels by the cricoid cartilage. Level VI nodes, the paratracheal nodes, are in the visceral or central compartment of the neck. This compartment extends from the hyoid bone superiorly to the suprasternal notch inferiorly. On each side of the neck, the lateral border of the central neck compartment is formed by the medial border of the carotid sheath. Level VII nodes are in the superior mediastinum (**Fig. 1**).

---

[a] Department of Radiology, University of Pennsylvania School of Medicine, Hospital of the University of Pennsylvania, 3400 Spruce Street, Philadelphia, PA 19104, USA
[b] Division of Endocrinology, Diabetes, and Metabolism, Department of Medicine, University of Pennsylvania School of Medicine, 700 CRB, 415 Curie Boulevard, Philadelphia, PA 19104, USA
* Corresponding author.
E-mail address: jill.langer@uphs.upenn.edu (J.E. Langer).

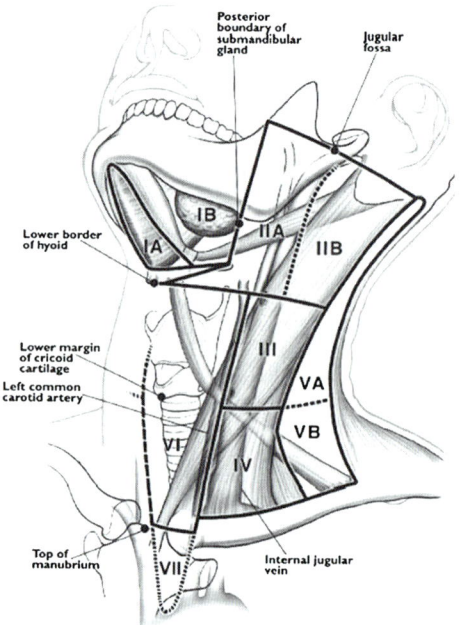

Fig. 1. Anatomic diagram of the lymph node levels of the neck established by The American Joint Committee on Cancer Staging and the American Academy of Otolaryngology–Head and Neck Surgery. This imaging-based classification system groups the cervical nodes by levels rather than surface anatomy. Levels I through V are located in the lateral compartment of the neck; levels VI and VII are located in the central neck compartment. (*From* Som PM, Curtin HD, Mancuso AA. An imaging-based classification for the cervical nodes designed as an adjunct to recent clinically based nodal classifications. Arch Otolaryngol Head Neck Surg 125:394; with permission. Copyright © 1999, American Medical Association. All rights reserved.)

TECHNIQUE

In general, higher-frequency, linear transducers offer the best spatial resolution, whereas lower frequencies give better tissue penetration of the emitted sound waves. Because the findings of metastatic thyroid cancer may be subtle, the examination should be performed with the highest frequency possible. The superficial neck nodes should be evaluated with a linear, high-frequency transducer of at least 7.5 MHz, preferably greater than 10 MHz.[14] Evaluation of the deep lymph nodes of the neck and the superior mediastinal nodes may require a lower frequency (5 to 7.5 MHz), small footprint curvilinear or sector probe that allows deeper sound penetration and can be positioned in the narrow suprasternal notch. Transducers with color Doppler capability are also preferred because assessment of the vascularity of lymph nodes is often helpful in identifying metastatic disease.

The patient should be in a supine position, with a pillow or rolled towel under the upper back to allow maximal extension of the neck. This technique is particularly important to examine the lower level IV and level VI nodes and the upper mediastinum. The examination should be systematic, imaging all the lymph node levels in the transverse plane. The longitudinal plane should also be used to examine levels II through V. Gray-scale sonography is used to identify the size, shape, and nodal architecture. Color Doppler sonography, or the more sensitive power Doppler sonography, is then performed to assess the presence and distribution of intranodular vessels.[15–18]

NORMAL LYMPH NODES

Normal cervical lymph nodes are typically imaged during high-frequency sonography examination of the neck. Normal nodes are most commonly seen in the submandibular region, the upper cervical chain, and the posterior triangle (Levels IB, II, III, and V, respectively).[19,20] There is a tendency for nodes to be larger with advancing age, perhaps because of increased fat deposition.[20] The normal node is typically flat, oval, or kidney bean shaped (**Fig. 2**). Nodes in the submandibular region and

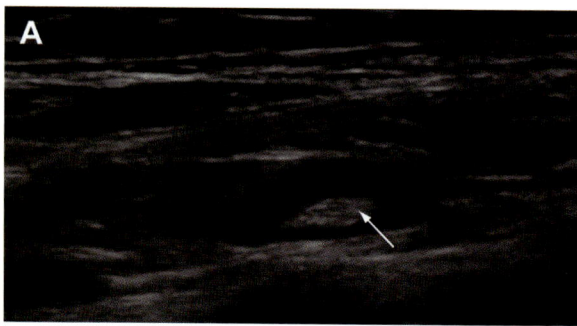
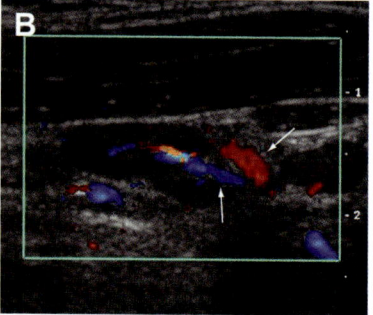

Fig. 2. Normal lateral cervical lymph nodes. (*A*) Sagittal view of a mid cervical lymph node (level III) demonstrates the sonographic appearance of a normal lymph node with a uniformly hypoechoic periphery and a central echogenic hilum (*arrow*). (*B*) Transverse color Doppler shows central vascularity within the feeding artery and vein (*arrow*) entering the hilum.

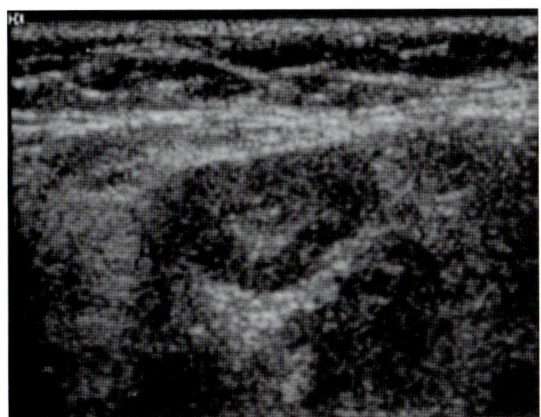

Fig. 3. Normal submandibular lymph node. Sagittal view of a submandibular (level IB) node demonstrates a rounded configuration but normal echogenic hilum. Although a rounded shape may raise concern for nodal pathology, submandibular nodes maybe rounded in the absence of pathology.

parotid region may be rounded without underlying pathology (**Fig. 3**). Each lymph node is encased in a dense connective tissue known as the capsule. The periphery of the lymph node is known as the cortex and contains most of the lymphoid follicles. This dominant portion of the lymph node is typically hypoechoic, less commonly isoechoic to the surrounding soft tissues.[14,19] The inner part of the node or the medulla is made up of fluid-filled sinuses and medullary cords from which the lymph flows from the afferent lymphatic vessels into the node. The feeding artery and vein are located in the hilum of the node along with the efferent draining lymphatic vessels.[15–17] On sonography, the central nodal hilus is typically an echogenic structure caused by sound reflecting off the multiple fluid-filled sinuses.[15,21,22] Normal nodes typically demonstrate only hilar vessels or are avascular, with the ability to detect vascularity by sonography paralleling the size of the node **Figure 2**.[15,16]

METASTATIC LYMPH NODES

Various sonographic features have been described to aid in the differentiation of metastatic lymph nodes from normal ones, including increased lymph node size, rounded shape, absence of the echogenic hilus, hyper echogenicity, cystic change, presence of calcifications, and increased vascularity. Cervical lymph node size is unreliable as the sole criterion of metastatic thyroid carcinoma because hyperplastic nodes may be large and metastatic nodes may be normal in size (**Fig. 4**).[7,23,24] In general, lymph nodes are considered to be enlarged when the short axis exceeds 8 mm in the submandibular region (Level II) and 5 mm in other cervical regions.[25,26] Malignant infiltration typically transforms nodes from an oval to a rounded shape (**Fig. 5**). This change in shape is quantified by an increase in the short axis/long axis (S:L) ratio to a value greater than 0.5 (**Figs. 5, 6**).[14,24,27,28] An elevated S:L ratio carries a false-positive rate of approximately 10% to 15%, however, reflecting the common occurrence of lateral cervical node enlargement attributable to benign inflammatory conditions of the oropharynx,[29,30] and a false-negative rate of 20% reflecting the propensity for microscopic nodal metastases to occur without enlarging the node, particularly with papillary thyroid carcinomas.[1,2]

Absence of the echogenic hilus of a lymph node raises concern for tumor infiltration, obliterating the central sinuses[14,21,31] and has been reported to carry a positive predictive value of 92% for the presence of metastatic thyroid cancer (see **Fig. 6**).[30] It is worth noting that the detection of a normal hilum does not exclude metastatic disease to that node.[14] The hilar vessels may still be

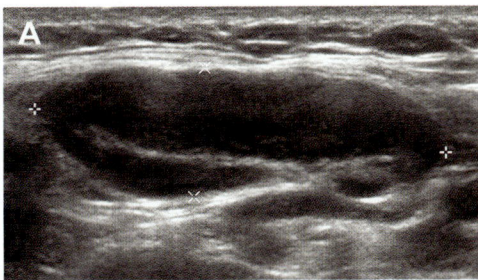
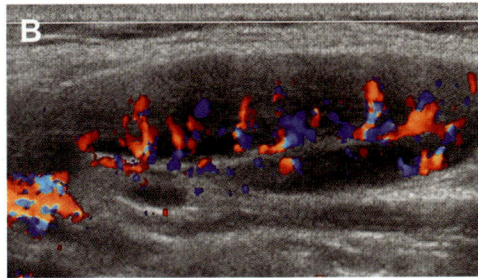

Fig. 4. Hyperplastic lymph node. (A) Sagittal gray-scale image of a 2.2 cm long level IIA node in a 22-year-old patient who had a history of thyroid cancer. Although the node is enlarged, the sonographic morphology was otherwise normal with a uniformly hypoechoic periphery and a regular, linear central echogenic hilum. (B) Color Doppler image of this node shows slightly increased central flow. Fine needle aspiration of this node demonstrated only reactive hyperplasia.

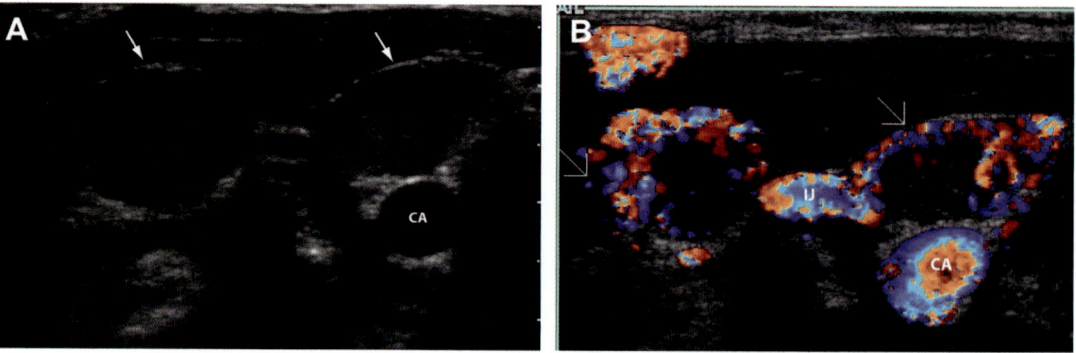

Fig. 5. Metastatic nodes with rounded shape. (A) Transverse view of the right lateral cervical chain shows two abnormal lymph nodes (arrows) that are rounded without a visible echogenic hilum. (B) Both nodes show marked periphery vascularity on color Doppler examination.

identified with color or power Doppler sonography even in the setting of a non-visualized hilum secondary to metastatic disease.[15,18] Malignant nodes may demonstrate abnormal vascular patterns, including increased peripheral or capsular flow either diffusely or focally, with or without increased central vascularity.[7,15] Tumor deposits within a node may displace hilar vessels, produce avascular areas, or demonstrate focal regions with tortuous and aberrant vessels.[15,18] These vascular patterns help to differentiate metastatic nodes from enlarged hyperplastic nodes, which tend to preserve nodal architecture with only increased central flow (see **Fig. 4**).

Hyperechogenicity, calcifications, and cystic change are features that highly predict the presence of metastatic thyroid cancer, particularly papillary thyroid cancer to affected nodes. Hyperechogenicity of a node relative to the adjacent musculature is a finding noted in up to 86% of metastatic lymph nodes from papillary thyroid cancer and is a rarely noted in benign nodes.[7,27,28,30] The increased echogenicity is believed to be secondary to malignant follicular cells and colloid deposition within the metastatic node, which alters the normal hypoechoic appearance of cortex to the increased echogenicity typical of thyroid tissue (**Fig. 7**).[30] Initially the metastatic tumor deposits may be noted as tiny, focal hyperechoic regions in the periphery of the node or near the hilum. The sonographic detection of these often subtle metastatic foci to otherwise normal-appearing nodes can be improved by the use of color Doppler examination, which demonstrates focal increased vascularity in the suspect areas (**Fig. 8**). As the node becomes progressively infiltrated with tumor, it demonstrates more diffuse regions of hyperechogenicity and increased vascularity, and typically other features of metastatic disease, such as enlarged size, rounded shape, obliteration of the hilum, calcifications, and cystic necrosis.[7]

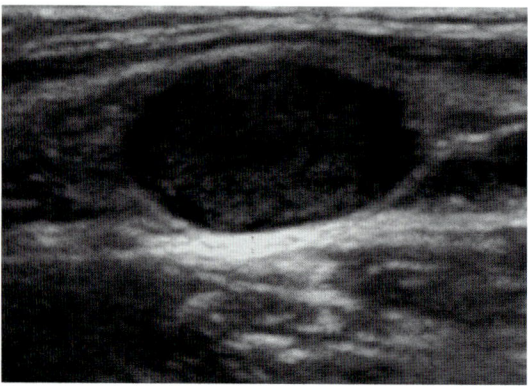

Fig. 6. Lack of the normal hilum. Sagittal view of a right lateral lymph node shows absence of the normal fatty hilum. Additionally this node is rounded in configuration and measured 8 × 14 mm for an S:L ratio of 0.57.

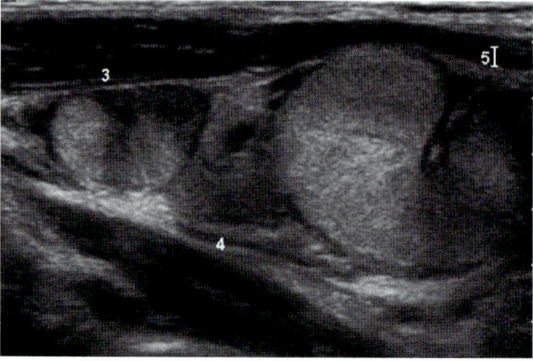

Fig. 7. Hyperechoic lymph nodes. Multiple enlarged and hyperechoic lateral cervical lymph nodes are seen (numbers 3–5) on this sagittal view of the left lateral neck in this 36-year-old patient who had metastatic follicular variant of papillary cancer.

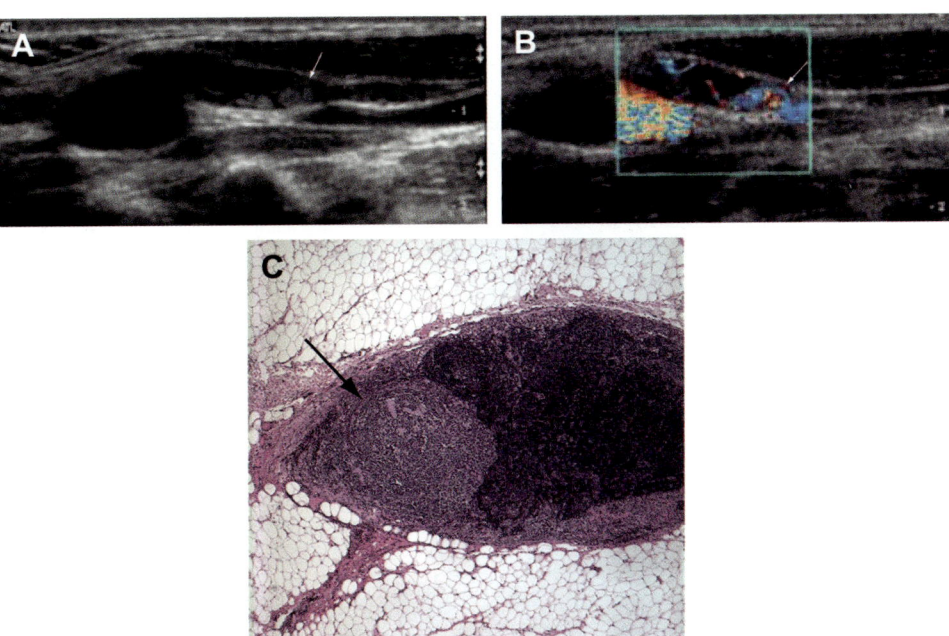

Fig. 8. Small hyperechoic foci. (*A*) Sagittal view of a lateral cervical lymph node demonstrates a subtle region of hyperechogenicity in the lower aspect of this node (*arrow*) corresponding to a small metastatic focus. (*B*) Color vascular examination shows focally increased flow in the same region (*arrow*). Fine needle aspiration of the focal area was positive for papillary thyroid carcinoma. (*C*) Pathology specimen obtained from a different patient shows a metastatic focus (*arrow*) of thyroid cancer within the periphery of the otherwise normal node. (*Courtesy of Dr Zubair Baloch, Philadelphia, PA.*)

Intranodal calcifications have been noted in 46% to 69% of metastatic nodes from papillary thyroid carcinoma (**Fig. 9**).[7,30,32] Although intranodal calcifications may be seen in nodes affected by tuberculosis, sarcoidosis, and following radiotherapy, they are rare in non-thyroid metastases.[27] The calcifications are typically fine or punctate and are located in the periphery of the node.[27,30]

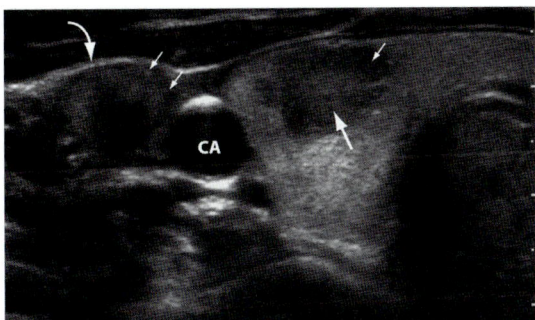

Fig. 9. Nodal calcifications. Transverse view of the right lobe of the thyroid shows a 1.5-cm papillary thyroid cancer (*large arrow*) that contains subtle punctuate microcalcifications (*small arrow*). A metastatic right lateral cervical lymph node (*curved arrow*) lateral to the carotid artery (CA) is also seen to contain these calcifications (*small arrows*).

Perhaps the most specific feature of metastatic papillary thyroid cancer is the tendency of these nodes to undergo cystic degeneration. Affected nodes may contain a small solitary cystic area or multiple scattered cystic areas, or may undergo near complete replacement of the parenchyma by cystic fluid.[7,27,33–35] Often another characteristic feature, such as calcifications, increased echogenicity, or increased vascularity, is noted with the solid component of partially cystic nodes (**Fig. 10**).[7] In some patients, particularly children, cystic nodal metastases may become large or may be the sole presentation of the underlying malignancy.[34,35] These cystic metastases should be differentiated from branchial cleft cysts, which are rare and tend to occur just medial to the border of the sternocleidomastoid muscle in the upper neck, whereas cystic nodes are more common in the lower neck. In confusing cases, aspiration of the lesion for cytologic evaluation and thyroglobulin assay is recommended.[29,33,34]

EVALUATION OF THE POST-THYROIDECTOMY BED

Following near-total thyroidectomy and remnant ablation, only a minimal amount of echogenic tissue, likely reflecting a combination of normal

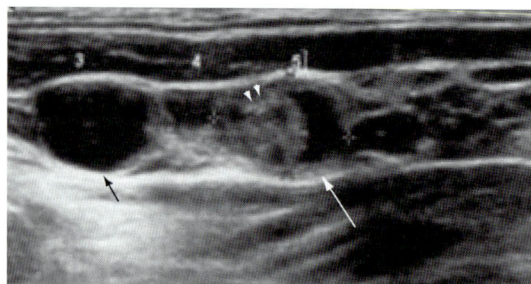

Fig. 10. Cystic nodes. Sagittal view of the right neck shows a chain of metastatic lymph nodes with varying degrees of cystic change. The most superior node (*short black arrow*) is nearly entirely cystic. The most inferior node (*long white arrow*) has both cystic regions and solid elements that contain calcifications.

connective tissue and scar tissue, is noted in the thyroidectomy bed (**Fig. 11**). Recurrent thyroid cancer in the bed typically appears as a solid or mixed cystic and solid soft tissue mass, often with marked vascularity (**Fig. 12**).[3,11,36] If large masses or posteriorly positioned masses are noted in the central compartment of the neck, cross-sectional imaging with CT or MR may be necessary to evaluate for invasive disease into the trachea, esophagus, retropharyngeal space, or skull base, because sonography is limited in evaluating these areas.[29,37] Following thyroidectomy, metastatic disease to the paratracheal lymph nodes can be detected by identifying enlarged, cystic, calcified, or vascular paratracheal lymph nodes (**Figs. 13** and **14**).

MIMICS OF RECURRENT DISEASE

Various benign soft tissue findings may be noted in the postoperative neck that may be confused with

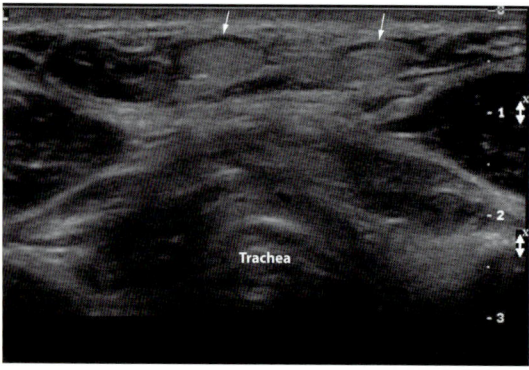

Fig. 11. Normal thyroidectomy bed. Transverse image at the level of the thyroid cartilage shows a small amount of heterogeneous soft tissue in the thyroidectomy bed. There are echogenic areas in the overlying musculature (*arrow*) consistent with expected postoperative change.

metastatic disease. Often the sternocleidomastoid muscle is partially resected causing it to have irregular echogenic regions representing scar often with fatty atrophy. The geometric shape, absence of vascular flow, and location of the echogenic areas in the muscle belly may be helpful features in minimizing concern that the soft tissue abnormalities reflect recurrent disease (see **Fig. 11**).

Other benign focal nonmalignant soft tissue lesions detected by sonography include foreign body granulomas and postoperative neuromas.[38,39] Granulomas may form in the operative bed because of foreign body reaction to suture material or as a nonspecific inflammatory response.[39] Some may have a characteristic appearance of a hypoechoic solid lesion with central curvilinear lines representing the suture material or a complex cystic lesion.[38,39] These granulomas are typically avascular or may be minimally vascular in the periphery and often are relatively superficial in location or within the sternocleidomastoid muscle (**Fig. 15**). Some granulomas require fine needle aspiration (FNA) to exclude a postoperative abscess or recurrence.

Approximately 1% to 2% of patients may develop a traumatic neuroma following neck dissection. Typically these are firm subcutaneous nodules located near the second cranial nerve.[40] About 40% of patients note characteristic sensitivity or pain during palpation of the lesion; in others, the diagnosis is presumptively established when exquisite pain is produced during attempted biopsy to exclude malignancy. These lesions tend to be long and narrow (low S:L ratio) and are solid with minimal vascularity. Similar to granulomas, they often have a central hyperechoic focus, which corresponds to dense collagenous material. Another feature that is helpful in the distinction of these lesions from lymphadenopathy is the their location posterior to but not immediately adjacent to the carotid artery (**Fig. 16**).[40]

The cervical esophagus, which lies posterior to the thyroid, or a pharyngoesophageal diverticulum, which most commonly occurs at the level of thyroid, may be noted during neck sonography.[41,42] Although air within the esophagus may be echogenic with shadowing and simulate a calcified lesion, the real-time examination demonstrates these foci to be mobile pockets of air within the esophagus particularly during swallowing (**Fig. 17**).

ULTRASOUND-GUIDED FINE NEEDLE ASPIRATION

Ultrasound-guided FNA of abnormal-appearing lymph nodes or other soft tissue abnormalities in the neck may be necessary to document the

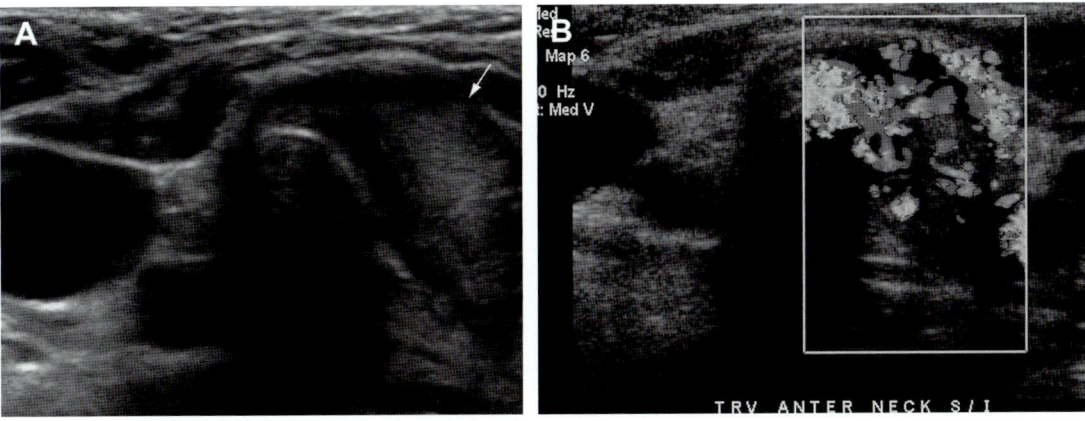

Fig. 12. Central neck recurrence. (A) Transverse image of the thyroidectomy bed shows a hypoechoic soft tissue mass (arrow) in the left bed representing recurrence at the site of tumor resection in this 42-year-old who had positive tumor margins. (B) Color Doppler image shows marked vascularity within the mass.

presence of metastatic disease to one or more compartments of the neck. Ultrasound-guided FNA is typically performed with a 25-gauge needle using real-time ultrasound monitoring and aseptic technique, similar to FNA of thyroid nodules.[43] One or more passes can be performed into the node targeting the most suspicious-appearing region. The reported sensitivities for this technique range from 80% to 90%.[44,45] Nondiagnostic aspirates are most common in predominantly cystic nodes and those with a small burden of metastatic disease. In these patients, the sample can be analyzed for the presence of thyroglobulin, a protein produced only by thyroid tissue and most thyroid cancers. The presence of thyroglobulin within an FNA specimen the presence of metastatic disease to that node.[46]

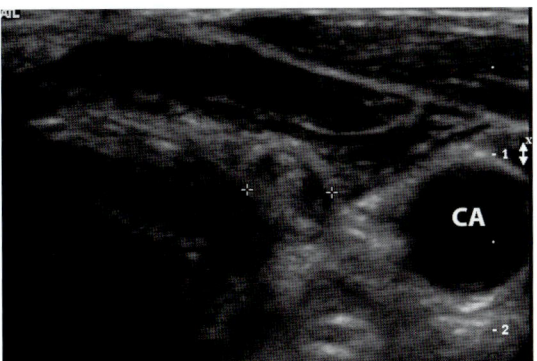

Fig. 13. Recurrence to a paratracheal lymph node. A calcified 5-mm lymph node, surgically proved to be a metastatic paratracheal node, was the only region of recurrence in this 37-year-old woman. CA, common carotid artery.

CLINICAL SCENARIOS FOR ULTRASOUND LYMPH NODE EVALUATION
Preoperatively

Imaging of the neck before surgery for thyroid carcinoma is necessary to determine the appropriate extent of surgical resection. In patients who present with symptoms such as hoarseness, airway compromise, or a rapidly enlarging neck mass, cross-sectional imaging may be necessary to assess for invasion of the tumor into the trachea, esophagus, and adjacent soft tissue structures.[37] Fortunately the vast majority of patients have less aggressive lesions that are confined to the thyroid or have limited extension into the adjacent soft tissue, often with regional lymph node metastases. Sonography has been established as the most sensitive imaging test to diagnose these nodal metastases.[3–7]

At initial diagnosis of differentiated thyroid cancer (DTC), up to 30% of patients have lymph node metastases detected by palpation or imaging.[47,48] Lymph node metastases are noted in up to 60% of patients on histologic review in centers performing ipsilateral and central neck dissections in all patients.[1,8,49] Palpation alone of the lateral neck compartments is not adequate and does not substitute for sonographic evaluation. Although the thyroid itself limits sonographic visualization of central neck lymph nodes before thyroidectomy, the lateral neck compartments can be assessed. In a recent series, ultrasound evaluation identified nonpalpable lateral compartment lymph nodes in 14% of patients undergoing initial surgery.[10] Even when lymph nodes were palpable, sonographic assessment of the extent of lymph node involvement altered 40% of the operative procedures by changing the extent of

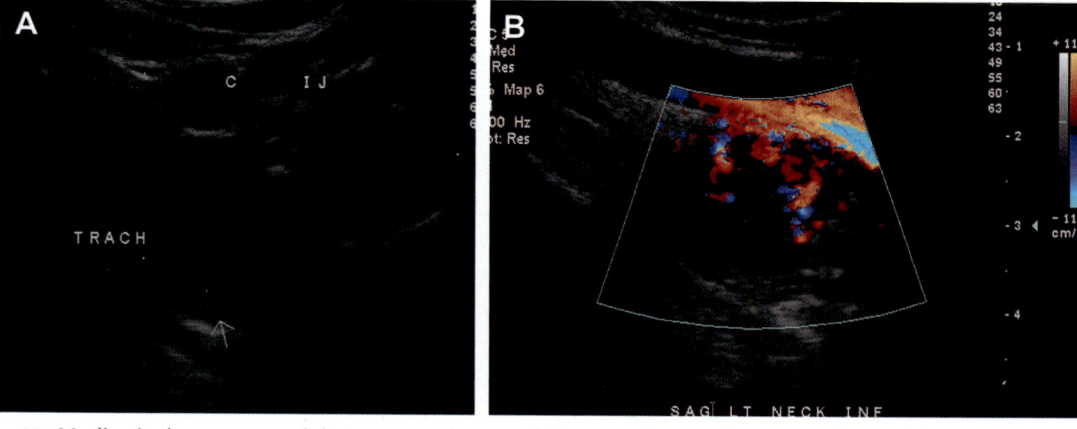

Fig. 14. Mediastinal recurrence. (*A*) Transverse image of the superior mediastinum obtained by using a curved 8-MHz transducer in the suprasternal notch detected this 2-cm soft tissue mass immediately adjacent to the trachea. (*B*) Sagittal color image demonstrates marked vascularity to this metastatic level VII node. C, carotid artery; IJ, internal jugular vein.

resection.[9,10] At the time of initial surgery, metastatic lateral lymph nodes are usually located ipsilateral to the primary tumor.[1,8] In fact, if a cancer is unilateral, it is unusual (18%) to have contralateral involvement of the lateral neck compartment.[1] Modified lateral neck dissection in these patients who have clinical (palpation or ultrasound) evidence of lateral lymph node metastases improves survival.[48] Before thyroidectomy, therefore, sonographic evaluation of the lateral compartment and the central compartment as limited by the thyroid is recommended by the recently published guidelines of the American Thyroid Association and the American Association of Clinical Endocrinologists.[50,51]

Surveillance for Recurrent Disease

The primary goal of follow-up in patients who have DTC is the early discovery of recurrent disease. The overall risk for local recurrence of papillary thyroid cancer, either in cervical lymph nodes or in the thyroid bed, is up to 30%.[47] Most recurrences appear in the first decade after initial therapy; however, a small number emerge decades after diagnosis.

In the past, a radioiodine whole-body scan was considered the main tool for disease detection during surveillance, but this has recently been discredited because of failure to identify metastatic lymph nodes even when documented by ultrasound.[52] For patients who have undetectable

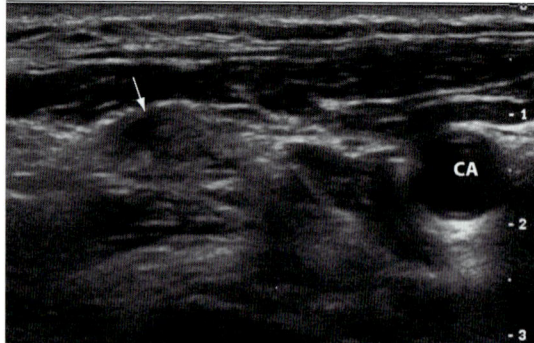

Fig. 15. Foreign body granuloma. Transverse image of the left neck showed this soft tissue lesion with a markedly echogenic central focus in the superficial tissues of the left neck (*marked by electronic calipers*). Although the fine needle aspiration was negative for malignancy, the patient underwent resection of this lesion, which proved to be a granuloma.

Fig. 16. Posttraumatic neuromas. Transverse image of the right lateral neck in a 53-year-old man who had a history of papillary thyroid cancer and previous right lateral neck dissection shows a heterogeneous soft tissue abnormality (*arrow*) remote from the carotid artery (CA). The patient experienced a sharp and radiating pain when FNA was attempted. It has been stable for more than 4 years and is presumed neuroma.

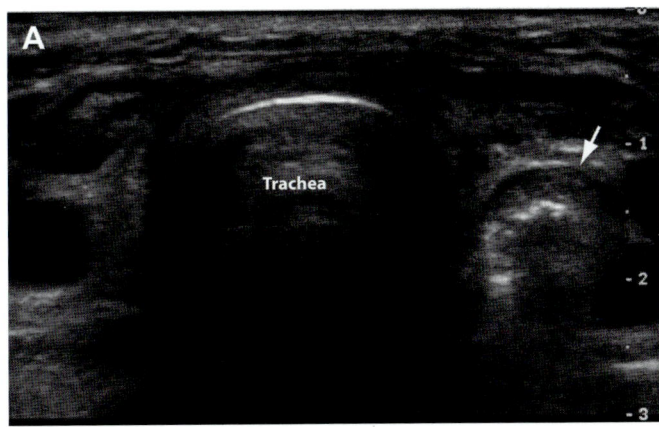 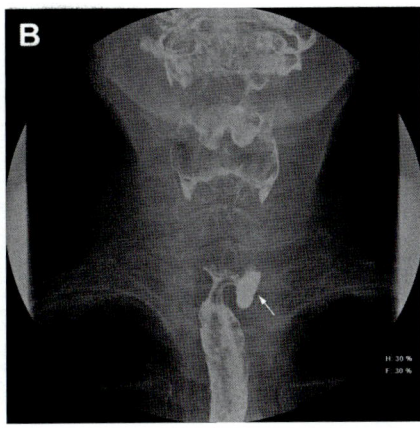

Fig. 17. Esophageal diverticulum. (A) Transverse view of the neck in a 70-year-old woman who had an undetectable serum thyroglobulin 3 years after thyroidectomy. A rounded, air-containing soft tissue structure was noted just lateral to the trachea (arrow). (B) Frontal radiograph from a barium swallow confirms the presence of an esophageal diverticulum immediately adjacent to the trachea.

serum thyroglobulin levels on levothyroxine suppression, the combination of a detectable stimulated serum thyroglobulin level with neck sonography identifies 95% of patients who have metastatic lymph nodes and has a negative predictive value of 99%.[5,53,54] The American Thyroid Association guidelines therefore support the use of only stimulated thyroglobulin and cervical ultrasound rather than the use of radioiodine scanning for surveillance in low-risk patients who have DTC.[50]

The timing and interval for performance of neck ultrasound depend on the risk status of the patient. The American Thyroid Association DTC guidelines suggest that "cervical ultrasound to evaluate the thyroid bed and central and lateral cervical nodal compartments should be performed at 6 and 12 months and then annually for at least 3 to 5 years, depending on the patient's risk for recurrent disease and thyroglobulin status."[50] If the serum thyroglobulin level remains detectable and other structural body imaging is negative, cervical ultrasound should continue to be done on regular interval. If the stimulated serum thyroglobulin level is undetectable and a cervical ultrasound is negative, however, the usefulness of subsequent ultrasound imaging is low.[55]

The distribution of persistent or recurrent lymph node metastases is most commonly the central compartment (35%–50%), followed by the ipsilateral lateral neck (20%–30%). Only rarely (8%–15%) is the contralateral lateral neck area involved.[8,9] Within the levels of the lateral neck, a recent study reported that the pattern of metastatic lymph node involvement was 50% for levels II and III, 40% for level IV, and only 20% for level V.[56] Palpation is insensitive for detection of recurrent or residual disease and sonographic identification of nonpalpable metastatic lymph nodes alters the extent of surgical resection in up to 70% of patients undergoing reoperation.[9,10]

SUMMARY

Sonography has been established as the most sensitive imaging modality to assess the neck for metastatic thyroid carcinoma. Lymph node metastases may vary from subtle alterations in echogenicity or vascular patterns to more obvious findings of calcifications and cystic changes within an affected node. Identification of metastatic disease by sonography may affect the extent of surgical resection at the time of diagnosis. Sonographic surveillance and sonographic-guided FNA offers to the ability to detect and document early thyroid cancer recurrence in the neck.

REFERENCES

1. Mirallie E, Visset J, Sagan C, et al. Localization of cervical node metastasis of papillary thyroid carcinoma. World J Surg 1999;23(9):970–3 [discussion: 973–74].
2. Mazzaferri EL, Kloos RT. Clinical review 128: current approaches to primary therapy for papillary and follicular thyroid cancer. J Clin Endocrinol Metab 2001; 86(4):1447–63.
3. Antonelli A, Miccoli P, Ferdeghini M, et al. Role of neck ultrasonography in the follow-up of patients operated on for thyroid cancer. Thyroid 1995;5(1):25–8.
4. Schlumberger M, Berg G, Cohen O, et al. Follow-up of low-risk patients with differentiated thyroid

carcinoma: a European perspective. Eur J Endocrinol 2004;150(2):105–12.
5. Torlontano M, Attard M, Crocetti U, et al. Follow-up of low risk patients with papillary thyroid cancer: role of neck ultrasonography in detecting lymph node metastases. J Clin Endocrinol Metab 2004;89(7): 3402–7.
6. Torlontano M, Crocetti U, Augello G, et al. Comparative evaluation of recombinant human thyrotropin-stimulated thyroglobulin levels, 131I whole-body scintigraphy, and neck ultrasonography in the follow-up of patients with papillary thyroid microcarcinoma who have not undergone radioiodine therapy. J Clin Endocrinol Metab 2006;91(1):60–3.
7. Leboulleux S, Girard E, Rose M, et al. Ultrasound criteria of malignancy for cervical lymph nodes in patients followed up for differentiated thyroid cancer. J Clin Endocrinol Metab 2007;92(9):3590–4.
8. Machens A, Hinze R, Thomusch O, et al. Pattern of nodal metastasis for primary and reoperative thyroid cancer. World J Surg 2002;26(1):22–8.
9. Kouvaraki MA, Shapiro SE, Fornage BD, et al. Role of preoperative ultrasonography in the surgical management of patients with thyroid cancer. Surgery 2003;134(6):946–55.
10. Stulak JM, Grant CS, Farley DR, et al. Value of preoperative ultrasonography in the surgical management of initial and reoperative papillary thyroid cancer. Arch Surg 2006;141(5):489–96.
11. Sutton RT, Reading CC, Charboneau JW, et al. US-guided biopsy of neck masses in postoperative management of patients with thyroid cancer. Radiology 1988;168(3):769–72.
12. Som PM, Curtin HD, Mancuso AA. An imaging-based classification for the cervical nodes designed as an adjunct to recent clinically based nodal classifications. Arch Otolaryngol Head Neck Surg 1999; 125(4):388–96.
13. Som PM, Curtin HD, Mancuso AA. Imaging-based nodal classification for evaluation of neck metastatic adenopathy. AJR Am J Roentgenol 2000;174(3): 837–44.
14. Vassallo P, Wernecke K, Roos N, et al. Differentiation of benign from malignant superficial lymphadenopathy: the role of high-resolution US. Radiology 1992; 183(1):215–20.
15. Ahuja A, Ying M, King A, et al. Lymph node hilus: gray scale and power Doppler sonography of cervical nodes. J Ultrasound Med 2001;20(9):987–92, quiz 994.
16. Ying M, Ahuja A, Brook F, et al. Power Doppler sonography of normal cervical lymph nodes. J Ultrasound Med 2000;19(8):511–7.
17. Ahuja AT, Ying M, Ho SS, et al. Distribution of intranodal vessels in differentiating benign from metastatic neck nodes. Clin Radiol 2001;56(3): 197–201.
18. Wu CH, Chang YL, Hsu WC, et al. Usefulness of Doppler spectral analysis and power Doppler sonography in the differentiation of cervical lymphadenopathies. AJR Am J Roentgenol 1998;171(2): 503–9.
19. Ying M, Ahuja A, Brook F, et al. Sonographic appearance and distribution of normal cervical lymph nodes in a Chinese population. J Ultrasound Med 1996;15(6):431–6.
20. Ying M, Ahuja A, Brook F. Sonographic appearances of cervical lymph nodes: variations by age and sex. J Clin Ultrasound 2002;30(1):1–11.
21. Rubaltelli L, Proto E, Salmaso R, et al. Sonography of abnormal lymph nodes in vitro: correlation of sonographic and histologic findings. AJR Am J Roentgenol 1990;155(6):1241–4.
22. Bruneton JN, Balu-Maestro C, Marcy PY, et al. Very high frequency (13 MHz) ultrasonographic examination of the normal neck: detection of normal lymph nodes and thyroid nodules. J Ultrasound Med 1994;13(2):87–90.
23. van den Brekel MW, Stel HV, Castelijns JA, et al. Cervical lymph node metastasis: assessment of radiologic criteria. Radiology 1990;177(2):379–84.
24. Ying M, Ahuja A, Metreweli C. Diagnostic accuracy of sonographic criteria for evaluation of cervical lymphadenopathy. J Ultrasound Med 1998;17(7): 437–45.
25. Bruneton JN, Roux P, Caramella E, et al. Ear, nose, and throat cancer: ultrasound diagnosis of metastasis to cervical lymph nodes. Radiology 1984;152(3): 771–3.
26. Ying M, Ahuja A. Sonography of neck lymph nodes. Part I: normal lymph nodes. Clin Radiol 2003;58(5): 351–8.
27. Ahuja A, Ying M. Sonography of neck lymph nodes. Part II: abnormal lymph nodes. Clin Radiol 2003; 58(5):359–66.
28. Ahuja AT, Chow L, Chick W, et al. Metastatic cervical nodes in papillary carcinoma of the thyroid: ultrasound and histological correlation. Clin Radiol 1995;50(4):229–31.
29. Gor DM, Langer JE, Loevner LA. Imaging of cervical lymph nodes in head and neck cancer: the basics. Radiol Clin North Am 2006;44(1):101–10, viii.
30. Rosario PW, de Faria S, Bicalho L, et al. Ultrasonographic differentiation between metastatic and benign lymph nodes in patients with papillary thyroid carcinoma. J Ultrasound Med 2005;24(10):1385–9.
31. Chan BK, Desser TS, McDougall IR, et al. Common and uncommon sonographic features of papillary thyroid carcinoma. J Ultrasound Med 2003;22(10): 1083–90.
32. Kuna SK, Bracic I, Tesic V, et al. Ultrasonographic differentiation of benign from malignant neck lymphadenopathy in thyroid cancer. J Ultrasound Med 2006;25(12):1531–7, quiz 1538–40.

33. Kessler A, Rappaport Y, Blank A, et al. Cystic appearance of cervical lymph nodes is characteristic of metastatic papillary thyroid carcinoma. J Clin Ultrasound 2003;31(1):21–5.
34. Wunderbaldinger P, Harisinghani MG, Hahn PF, et al. Cystic lymph node metastases in papillary thyroid carcinoma. AJR Am J Roentgenol 2002;178(3):693–7.
35. Verge J, Guixa J, Alejo M, et al. Cervical cystic lymph node metastasis as first manifestation of occult papillary thyroid carcinoma: report of seven cases. Head Neck 1999;21(4):370–4.
36. Simeone JF, Daniels GH, Hall DA, et al. Sonography in the follow-up of 100 patients with thyroid carcinoma. AJR Am J Roentgenol 1987;148(1):45–9.
37. King AD, Ahuja AT, To EW, et al. Staging papillary carcinoma of the thyroid: magnetic resonance imaging vs ultrasound of the neck. Clin Radiol 2000;55(3):222–6.
38. Gritzmann N, Hollerweger A, Macheiner P, et al. Sonography of soft tissue masses of the neck. J Clin Ultrasound 2002;30(6):356–73.
39. Langer JE, Luster E, Horii SC, et al. Chronic granulomatous lesions after thyroidectomy: imaging findings. AJR Am J Roentgenol 2005;185(5):1350–4.
40. Yabuuchi H, Kuroiwa T, Fukuya T, et al. Traumatic neuroma and recurrent lymphadenopathy after neck dissection: comparison of radiologic features. Radiology 2004;233(2):523–9.
41. Mercer D, Blachar A, Khafif A, et al. Real-time sonography of Killian-Jamieson diverticulum and its differentiation from thyroid nodules. J Ultrasound Med 2005;24(4):557–60.
42. Kwak JY, Kim EK. Sonographic findings of Zenker diverticula. J Ultrasound Med 2006;25(5):639–42.
43. Takashima S, Sone S, Nomura N, et al. Nonpalpable lymph nodes of the neck: assessment with US and US-guided fine-needle aspiration biopsy. J Clin Ultrasound 1997;25(6):283–92.
44. Frasoldati A, Valcavi R. Challenges in neck ultrasonography: lymphadenopathy and parathyroid glands. Endocr Pract 2004;10(3):261–8.
45. Boi F, Baghino G, Atzeni F, et al. The diagnostic value for differentiated thyroid carcinoma metastases of thyroglobulin (Tg) measurement in washout fluid from fine-needle aspiration biopsy of neck lymph nodes is maintained in the presence of circulating anti-Tg antibodies. J Clin Endocrinol Metab 2006;91(4):1364–9.
46. Cignarelli M, Ambrosi A, Marino A, et al. Diagnostic utility of thyroglobulin detection in fine-needle aspiration of cervical cystic metastatic lymph nodes from papillary thyroid cancer with negative cytology. Thyroid 2003;13(12):1163–7.
47. Schlumberger M. Papillary and follicular thyroid carcinoma. N Engl J Med 1998;338:297–306.
48. Noguchi S, Maurakami N, Yamashita H, et al. Papillary thyroid carcinoma: modified radical neck dissection improves prognosis. Arch Surg 1998;133:276–80.
49. Ito Y, Tomoda C, Uruno T, et al. Ultrasonographically and anatomopathologically detectable node metastases in the lateral compartment as indicators of wrose relapse-free survival in patients with papillary thyroid carcinoma. World J Surg 2005;29:917–20.
50. Cooper DS, Doherty GM, Haugen BR, et al. Management guidelines for patients with thyroid nodules and differentiated thyroid cancer. Thyroid 2006;16(2):109–42.
51. American Association of Clinical Endocrinologists and Associazone Medici Endocrinologi medical guidelines for clinical practice for the diagnosis and management of thyroid nodules. Endocr Pract 2006;12:63–99.
52. Mazzaferri EL, Kloos RT. Is diagnostic iodine-131 scanning with recombinant human TSH useful in the follow-up of differentiated thyroid cancer after thyroid ablation. J Clin Endocrinol Metab 2002;87:1490–8.
53. Frasoldati A, Pesent M, Gallo M, et al. Diagnosis of neck recurrences in patients with differentiated thyroid carcinoma. Cancer 2003;97:90–6.
54. Pacini F, Molinaro E, Castagna MG, et al. Recombinant human thyrotropin-stimulated serum thyroglobulin combined with neck ultrasonography has the highest sensitivity in monitoring differentiated thyroid carcinoma. J Clin Endocrinol Metab 2003;88:3668–73.
55. Kloos RT, Mazzaferri EL. A single recombinant human thyrotropin-stimulated serum thyroglobulin measurement predicts differentiated thyroid carcinoma metastases three to five years later. J Clin Endocrinol Metab 2005;90(9):5047–57.
56. Kupferman ME, Patterson M, Mandel SJ, et al. Patterns of lateral neck metastasis in papillary thyroid carcinoma. Arch Otolaryngol Head Neck Surg 2004;130:857–60.

Surgical Approaches in Thyroid Cancer: What the Radiologist Needs to Know

Jason G. Newman, MD, FACS[a],*, Ara A. Chalian, MD[b],
Ashok R. Shaha, MD, FACS[c,d]

KEYWORDS

- Thyroid cancer treatment • Thyroid carcinoma
- Surgery for thyroid cancer • Management of thyroid cancer

According to several studies, the incidence of thyroid nodules is anywhere from 50% to 70% in the adult population,[1,2] whereas the incidence of silent malignancy ranges between 3% and 5%. At the same time, the incidence of clinically evident thyroid cancers ranges from 0.5 to 10 cases per 100,000 people.[3] Most of the patients who have cancer have well-differentiated cancers, with an excellent long-term prognosis. Some patients have well-differentiated cancers with a poor prognosis, and some have other less common types of thyroid cancers. The challenge for the clinician is to identify the patients who have cancers, to treat them according to the extent and aggressiveness of their disease, and to limit morbidity and mortality as much as possible.

ETIOLOGY OF THYROID CANCER

An increase in the incidence of thyroid cancer has been associated with exposure to ionizing radiation. This association has been demonstrated most profoundly in the Ukraine, after the Chernobyl nuclear reactor disaster in 1986. Ongoing studies from this region have shown an increased incidence of thyroid nodules and cancer in these populations, with a 7 to 15 year latency in general.[4,5]

An increased risk for thyroid carcinoma among women suggests a possible role for hormones in increasing the risk, but no such link has been definitely identified. Studies have also investigated the role of radioactivity from I131 in increasing the risk for thyroid cancer, but to date have concluded that it does not increase the risk. Countries with iodine deficiency have a higher incidence of follicular thyroid cancers compared with non–iodine-deficient countries, but the cause is unclear.[6]

There are certain genetic syndromes that increase the risk for thyroid cancer, or are associated with thyroid cancer, especially medullary thyroid cancer, which has been linked to several specific genetic abnormalities. In some cases, papillary thyroid cancer follows a familial pattern also. Several rare genetic disorders, including Cowden disease, multiple endocrine neoplasia (MEN), and Gardner syndrome, are also associated with a higher incidence of thyroid cancer.

EPIDEMIOLOGY OF THYROID CANCER

Over the last several decades, the incidence of thyroid cancer has increased dramatically. It is

---

[a] Department of Otorhinolaryngology, Head and Neck Surgery, Center for Cranial Base Surgery, University of Pennsylvania, Pennsylvania Hospital, 811 Spruce Street, Philadelphia, PA 19107, USA
[b] Department of Otorhinolaryngology: Head and Neck Surgery, University of Pennsylvania Medical Center, 3400 Spruce Street, 5th Floor Ravdin Building, Philadelphia, PA 19104, USA
[c] Memorial Sloan-Kettering Cancer Center, 1275 York Avenue, New York, NY 10065, USA
[d] Cornell University Medical College, New York, New York, USA
* Corresponding author.
E-mail address: Jason.newman@uphs.upenn.edu (J.G. Newman).

unclear if this increased incidence is real or if it may be attributable to more sensitive diagnostic techniques. Autopsy studies have shown that up to 30% of adults have incidental cancers smaller than 1cm at the time of death.[7] This finding may imply that our more sensitive methods of detecting cancers may not affect overall prognosis. According to the SEER database, there are approximately 37,340 people who will be diagnosed with thyroid cancer in the United States in 2008. Approximately 1530 people will die of thyroid cancer during the same year. The average age of diagnosis is 47 years, and the average age of death is 74 years. (NCI SEER Cancer Statistics Review).

The most common type of thyroid cancer is papillary thyroid cancer (PTC). It represents approximately 70% of thyroid cancers. Follicular thyroid carcinoma (FTC) represents approximately 15% of cancers and in combination with PTC composes the category of well-differentiated thyroid carcinomas (WDTC). Grouped into the less common cancers are medullary (4%–6%), anaplastic (3%–4%), and others (up to 5%). This group may include lymphoma, sarcoma, squamous cell carcinoma, and metastases.

EMBRYOLOGY OF THE THYROID GLAND

The thyroid gland has two separate sites of origin embryologically. Most of the gland is derived from endodermal anlage of the primitive gastrointestinal tract. The parafollicular, or C cells, are derived from the ectodermal neural crest. The thyroid descends from the region of the foramen cecum to rest in its normal anatomic position, just beneath the cricoid and along the anterior and lateral surfaces of the upper trachea.

Understanding the embryology of the thyroid gives an appreciation of the many abnormalities that can be seen in children and adults when the migration of the thyroid is incomplete. As the thyroid descends, it normally loses its attachment to the tongue at the foramen cecum when the thyroglossal duct fibroses. The thyroglossal duct may remain patent and remain lined with a ciliated pseudostratified epithelium. This phenomenon can lead to the midline thyroglossal duct cyst, which can be located anywhere between the normal anatomic location of the thyroid and the base of the tongue.

The descent of the thyroid into its normal anatomic position is profoundly affected by the heart, and as such, aberrant thyroid tissue can be found in many locations in the neck and mediastinum. Locations, including the esophagus, the larynx, the trachea, the lateral cervical lymph nodes, the pericardium, the aortic arch, and the base of tongue, have been well documented. A lingual (base of tongue) location of the thyroid may represent the only undescended thyroid tissue in the body (Fig. 1).

ANATOMY OF THE THYROID GLAND

The thyroid consists of two lateral lobes, an isthmus, and, in about one third of patients, a pyramidal lobe. The average gland weighs between 15 and 25 g. The gland sits over the midline of the trachea, and is attached to the cricoid and tracheal wall by a ligament of Berry, which represents condensations of the deep cervical and pretracheal fascia. The inferior border of the gland varies in location, but can be below or above the sternal notch.

The arterial supply to the gland is derived from two separate paired vessels. The inferior thyroid vessels come directly off of the thyrocervical trunk and enter the thyroid at approximately the midsection of the lateral lobe. They tend to supply both the superior and the inferior parathyroids. The superior thyroid arteries come off the carotid, usually as the first branch of the external carotid, but sometimes off the common carotid. Rarely, a small artery or pair of arteries may come directly from the aorta or brachiocephalic trunk, named the thyroid ima.

There are three main paired veins that drain the thyroid. There is some variability in location and presence, but they generally drain into the internal jugular veins and innominate vein.

The lymphatics of the thyroid consist of intraglandular and extraglandular components.

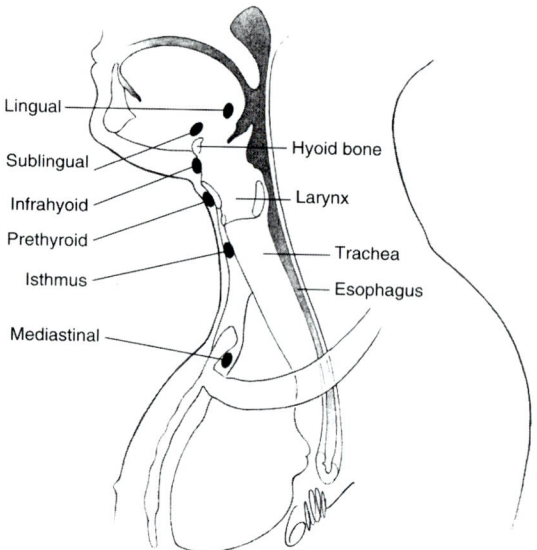

Fig. 1. Some common sites for midline ectopic thyroid masses. (From Randolph G. Surgery of the thyroid and parathyroid glands. Philadelphia: Elsevier Science; 2002. p. 13; with permission.)

Extraglandular lymphatics generally follow venous flow. The inferior portions of the lateral lobes drain along the tracheoesophageal groove into the central neck. The superior parts of the lobes drain toward the superior thyroid veins, and the isthmus may drain toward the delphian (prelaryngeal) lymph node or central neck nodes. More unusual, but clearly documented, are lymphatic pathways to the retropharyngeal region, accounting for metastases to the skull base. Based on clinical and anatomic review, the central lymphatics are generally considered the primary drainage pathways for thyroid cancers, with the lateral neck nodes being considered secondary levels of lymphatic spread. These facts are important from an imaging and a treatment perspective.

Two sets of nerves are intimately associated with the thyroid gland: the superior and the recurrent laryngeal nerves. They are branches of the 10th (vagus) cranial nerve. The recurrent laryngeal nerves have slightly different courses as they enter the larynx just under the thyroid gland. On the left, the nerve courses into the chest, around the aortic arch, and back up into the larynx. On the right, the nerve passes around the subclavian artery to course back up into the neck and into the larynx. Rarely, patients present with nonrecurrent laryngeal nerves. This presentation usually occurs on the right side, and is often associated with a retroesophageal subclavian artery. In rare cases of transposition of the great vessels, a left nonrecurrent nerve has been identified.

The parathyroid glands are also closely related to the thyroid anatomically. They tend to lie on the undersurface of the thyroid, and receive their blood supply from the inferior thyroid artery. Their anatomy is discussed in detail in another article in this issue.

ANATOMY OF THE NECK

The relevant anatomy of the neck for the thyroid surgeon and head and neck radiologist includes the entire anterior neck, from one trapezius muscle to the other, and from the base of skull to the mediastinum. Most important are the various lymphatic compartments of the neck, which have conventionally been divided into numbered compartments to aid in standardizing locations (**Fig. 2**). The lymphatics of the neck are divided into seven compartments. Level I includes the submental and submandibular nodes. They are located above the anterior and posterior bellies of the digastric muscle, which insert on the hyoid bone. This level is subdivided into level IA (submental), which is anterior to the digastric muscle, and level IB (submandibular), which is behind the

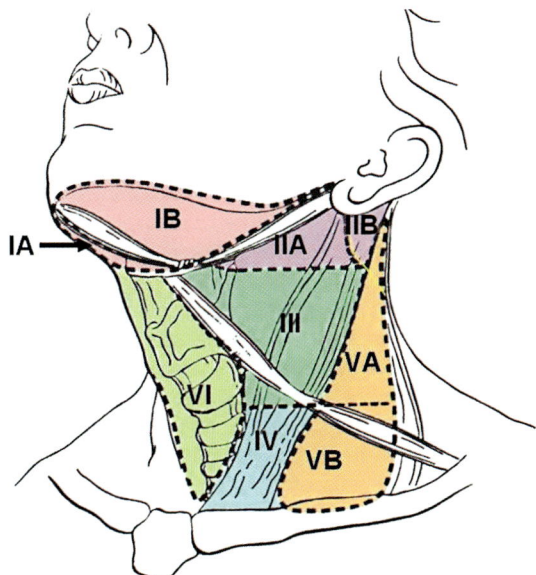

Fig. 2. Anatomy of the neck compartments. (*From* Harish K. Neck dissections: radical to conservative. World J Surg Oncol 2005;3:21; with permission.)

digastric. Levels II, II, and IV are all deep to the sternocleidomastoid muscle (SCM). The anterior and posterior border of all of these lymphatic groups is the anterior and posterior border of the SCM. Level II is the upper jugulodigastric group of nodes. Its superior boundary is the skull base, and its inferior boundary is at the level of the hyoid. It is subdivided by the 11th cranial nerve into an anterior (level IIA) and posterior (level IIB) compartment. Level III is the middle jugular nodal basin. Its inferior boundary is at the level of the cricoid. Level IV is the inferior jugular nodal basin. Its inferior boundary is the clavicle. Level V is the posterior triangle group of nodes. It lies between the posterior border of the SCM and the anterior border of the trapezius. Level VI is the anterior compartment, or central neck nodal basin. It is bordered laterally on both sides by the carotid sheath, superiorly by the hyoid, and inferiorly by the sternal notch. It is sometimes divided into the pretracheal (anterior to the trachea) and paratracheal (lateral to the trachea) compartments. Finally, Level VII is the anterior mediastinal compartment of nodes. It remains between the carotids, from the sternal notch to the level of the aortic arch, in the superior mediastinum.

Dissecting the lymph nodes to remove cancer or suspected cancer from patients who have thyroid abnormalities remains a mainstay in therapy. Determining which levels of the neck to dissect is greatly aided in many cases by the results of radiologic studies and understanding of the patterns of nodal metastasis. In cases of suspected pathologic adenopathy, it is helpful to include specific descriptors of a node's location. This description includes the anatomic level of the node and the relationship of the node to surrounding structures, such as the bifurcation of the carotid artery and the hyoid bone. Especially in cases of suspected cancer recurrence, this additional information is critical.

The pattern of spread of thyroid cancer to the lymph nodes is well documented. Initially, most thyroid cancers metastasize to the central compartment nodes (level VI). Several sentinel node studies have shown that in patients who have metastases, more than 80% are in the central neck.[8] Unfortunately, thyroid cancer often demonstrates "skip" metastases, making it hard to predict which levels of the neck will have metastatic nodes.[9,10] In large series, the lateral neck nodes are involved to varying degrees. Most commonly involved is level IV, followed by levels III, V, II, and I.[11] Level I nodal metastases are rare from thyroid cancer.

Contralateral metastases are most common in larger tumors, tumors that cross the midline, and recurrent cancers. The most commonly involved contralateral compartment is the paratracheal region. When this is positive, the risk for metastases to the lateral neck is higher.

There is significant controversy regarding if and when to dissect the lymph nodes in the neck, especially in necks without evidence of disease in the pretreatment setting. For this reason, it is especially important to thoroughly evaluate the thyroid itself and the central neck (as much as possible) and lateral neck in patients who have known or suspected thyroid cancers. Nodal metastasis, although common in thyroid cancer, has little prognostic implication in well-differentiated thyroid cancer.

STAGING OF THYROID CANCER

As with all cancers, staging systems for thyroid cancer not only help clarify and standardize reporting of these cancers but also attempt to predict prognosis and outcome. Several staging systems have been developed over time, using various factors to help stratify patients into higher and lower risk categories. One of the most widely accepted systems is the TNM staging. The T stage refers to the largest extent of tumor in the thyroid itself, the N to size and location of lymph nodes in the neck, and the M to the presence or absence of distant metastasis. Most staging systems, including the TNM, account for patient age in their determination of final stage, because of large studies that have shown the profound effect that age has on prognosis. The TNM staging has a cutoff of 45 years of age. Patients younger than age 45 who have any T stage and any N stage are still stage I, and even distant metastasis only places them in stage II. Older patients tend to have a poorer prognosis (**Fig. 3**). This staging system generally refers to WDTC only. Medullary, anaplastic, and other less common cancers are not accounted for in this staging.[12]

PATHOLOGY OF THYROID CANCER
Papillary Thyroid Cancer

Papillary thyroid cancer is the most common of thyroid cancers, but the true incidence is unknown, partly because of the often indolent nature of this cancer and because it often presents incidentally during workup or surgery for another diagnosis, or at the time of autopsy. Most patients diagnosed and treated for this cancer are either cured of the disease or live for many years after the diagnosis. Less than 50% of recurrences occur within the first 5 years, and it is not unusual for recurrences to present several decades after the initial diagnosis.[13]

Pathologically, this cancer resembles the cell from which it is derived, the follicular cell. It often retains the ability to concentrate iodine, secrete thyroglobulin, and even produce thyroid hormone. It often retains its ability to respond to thyrotropin (TSH) stimulation. Grossly, these tumors are poorly encapsulated, firm, and often have calcifications (psammoma bodies) within their substance. The presence of these calcifications is of diagnostic significance, because they are rarely present in other thyroid pathologies. These tumors, especially larger ones, may contain focal areas of hemorrhage and necrosis. PTC demonstrates papillary fronds along with follicular components. The nuclei have a characteristic appearance, with a feature described as "Orphan-Annie eyes" used to refer to the relatively empty appearance of the nucleoplasm.

Histologically, there are several variants of papillary thyroid carcinoma. Follicular variant of papillary thyroid carcinoma has a pattern of neoplastic follicles that are small with little colloid. They contain relatively fewer nuclear inclusions and psammoma bodies. The prognosis and biologic behavior is similar to that of papillary thyroid cancer. The tall cell variant of papillary thyroid carcinoma has neoplastic cells in which the height is twice the width. It is associated with more aggressive biologic characteristics and tends to metastasize earlier in its course. Overall, the prognosis is poor compared with classic papillary thyroid carcinoma.

Definition of TNM for Papillary and Follicular Carcinoma

Primary Tumor (T)

Note: All categories may be subdivided: (a) solitary tumor, (b) multifocal tumor (the largest determines the classification).

- TX Primary tumor cannot be assessed
- T0 No evidence of primary tumor
- T1 Tumor 2 cm or less in greatest dimension limited to the thyroid
- T2 Tumor more than 2 cm but not more than 4 cm in greatest dimension limited to the thyroid
- T3 Tumor more than 4 cm in greatest dimension limited to the thyroid or any tumor with minimal extrathyroid extension (e.g., extension to sternothyroid muscle or perithyroid soft tissue)
- T4a Tumor of any size extending beyond the thyroid capsule to invade subcutaneous soft tissues, larynx, trachea, esophagus, or recurrent laryngeal nerve
- T4b Tumor invades prevertebral fascia or encases carotid artery or mediastinal vessels

All anaplastic carcinomas are considered T4 tumors.

- T4a Intrathyroidal anaplastic carcinoma–surgically resectable
- T4b Extrathyroidal anaplastic carcinoma–surgically unresectable

Regional Lymph Nodes (N)

Regional lymph nodes are the central compartment, lateral cervical, and upper mediastinal lymph nodes.

- NX Regional lymph nodes cannot be assessed.
- N0 No regional lymph node metastatis
- N1 Regional lymph node metastatis
- N1a Metastasis to Level VI (pretracheal, paratracheal, and prelaryngeal/Delphian lymph nodes)
- N1b Metastasis to unilateral, bilateral, or contralateral cervical or superior mediastinal lymph nodes

Distant Metastasis (M)

- MX Distant metastasis cannot be assessed
- M0 No distant metastasis
- M1 Distant metastasis

STAGE GROUPING

Separate stage groupings are recommended for papillary or follicular, medullary, and anaplastic (undifferentiated) carcinoma.

Papillary or Follicular
Under 45 years

Stage I	Any T	Any N	M0
Stage II	Any T	Any N	M1

Papillary or Follicular
45 years and older

Stage I	T1	N0	M0
Stage II	T2	N0	M0
Stage III	T3	N0	M0
	T1	N1a	M0
	T2	N1a	M0
	T3	N1a	M0
Stage IVA	T4a	N0	M0
	T4a	N1a	M0
	T1	N1b	M0
	T2	N1b	M0
	T3	N1b	M0
	T4a	N1b	M0
Stage IVB	T4b	Any N	M0
Stage IVC	Any T	Any N	M1

Fig. 3. Staging of thyroid cancers. (*From* Greene FL, Page DL, Fleming ID, et al. AJCC Cancer staging manual. 6th edition. New York: Springer; 2002. p. 90–2. Used with permission of the American Joint Committee on Cancer (AJCC), Chicago, IL. The original source for this material is the AJCC Cancer Staging Manual, 6th edition (2002) published by Springer Science and Business Media, LLC, www.springerlink.com.)

It is common for PTC to demonstrate multifocal disease within the thyroid gland at the time of histologic examination. The incidence has been reported to be as high as 80% in the literature.[14,15] This fact has led to recommendations by many authors to consider total thyroidectomy at the time of initial presentation. They cite an incidence of recurrence of 5% to 20% in patients who have partial thyroid surgery.[15,16] Other authors, however, have demonstrated that locoregional recurrence does not affect long-term survival,[17,18] and thus they advocate less aggressive surgery to minimize morbidity in select patients.[19]

Extrathyroidal extension of the tumor has demonstrated prognostic significance, and thus helps determine extent of surgical and medical treatment.[20,21] Although the overlying strap muscles in the neck are the most commonly invaded structures, there are many cases of tracheal, laryngeal, esophageal, and other soft tissue extensions in the neck.

Regional metastasis to the neck and mediastinal lymph nodes is common for PTC. The published incidence varies from 40% to more than 75%, if one includes subclinical metastases[22,23] Abundant literature has investigated the role that regional metastasis has on prognosis, and there is no consensus. Although some studies have demonstrated a poorer prognosis for elderly patients who have nodal metastasis,[24,25] several studies have demonstrated that neck metastases do not adversely affect long-term survival or prognosis. A few have demonstrated that nodal metastasis improves prognosis, and still others suggest that the more nodes with metastasis, the better the prognosis.[13,15,26]

Age has proved to have prognostic significance in PTC and in other thyroid cancers. In general, younger age is associated with an improved prognosis.

Unlike regional metastasis, distant metastasis does seem to adversely affect prognosis. Approximately 10% of patients demonstrate metastasis to distant sites. Most commonly this involves the lungs, but the central nervous system and bones are common sites also. Studies have demonstrated that the volume of disease seems to affect prognosis, and macrometastases have been associated with almost a 50% 1-year rate of death.[27]

Follicular Thyroid Carcinoma

Follicular thyroid carcinoma (FTC) is the second most common type of thyroid cancer. It represents about 15% of thyroid cancers. Many authors have suggested that the prognosis is slightly poorer than that for papillary thyroid cancer, but others suggest that when matched for age and stage, the prognosis is similar. They contend that the differences in overall survival represent presentation of follicular cancers at later stages and in older patients in general. Grossly, on examination, these tumors are thickly encapsulated with focal necrosis and cystic changes.[28] The cells are small and monotonous. Psammoma bodies are rare, and the cells are organized into follicles that contain sparse colloid.

Both benign and malignant follicular lesions demonstrate follicular cells arranged in microfollicles, rosettes, or spindles, and thus they cannot be differentiated on fine needle aspiration. Capsular invasion is the only current method of distinguishing between the two. Because this can only be done once the entire capsule of the tumor has been evaluated histologically (unless gross invasion is visible before removal of the tumor), it is not uncommon for this diagnosis to be made after surgery.

Like PTC, FTC portends overall a good prognosis. In patients who have minimal capsular invasion, the prognosis is excellent, and few patients develop distant metastases or die of disease.[16,29,30] In patients who have capsular or vascular invasion, however, the prognosis is much worse. Similar to PTC, patients who have FTC do better at younger ages, and women may have a slightly better prognosis than men.

Clinically, follicular carcinomas tend to present with solitary thyroid mass. The incidence of multicentric disease within the thyroid is much lower than with PTC. Although the rate of regional lymphatic metastasis is low, presence of lymph nodes positive for follicular carcinoma is a poor prognostic indicator. The rate of local invasion into trachea, pharynx, and so forth, is higher in patients who have nodal metastases.[31]

Distant metastases are more common with FTC than with PTC. They tend to spread primarily to bone, and may present with pathologic fractures. These cancers also tend to spread to lung, liver, and brain. The prognosis is poor for patients who have distant metastasis.

Hürthle Cell Carcinoma

Hürthle cell carcinoma is a variant of follicular carcinoma. It accounts for 3% to 5% of thyroid cancers. It is composed of large acidophilic or oncocytic cells and does not generally take up radioiodine as well as classic follicular cancers. Like follicular carcinomas, the diagnosis can only be made after examination of the entire tumor capsule. The cancers generally have a slightly worse prognosis than other follicular carcinomas.[32,33] They are associated with a higher rate of lymph node and distant metastasis[23,34] than other follicular carcinomas.

Insular Thyroid Carcinoma

Although this cancer is listed as a variant of follicular thyroid carcinoma by the World Health Organization, it does not have many of the features associated with follicular or papillary thyroid cancers. Rare follicular structures are seen, and the cells may be arranged in trabeculae of cells surrounded by connective tissue.[35] Sometimes referred to as poorly differentiated carcinoma, this lesion has a poorer overall prognosis than other well-differentiated thyroid cancers. It is rare, and in limited studies it has demonstrated a 10-year mortality rate of 10% to 46%.[36–38]

Medullary Thyroid Carcinoma

Medullary thyroid carcinoma is unique among thyroid cancers in that it is derived from the parafollicular or C cells, which are a part of the amine precursor uptake and decarboxylation (APUD) cell system. These cells produce calcitonin and are unrelated to the iodine concentrating and thyroid hormone production of the gland. They are more closely related to other tumors of the neuroendocrine system, including carcinoid tumors and pheochromocytomas.

MTC is rare, and accounts for 3% to 5% of thyroid cancers. It comes in two forms, familial and sporadic. The familial form, which is less common than the sporadic form of MTC, is inherited as an autosomal dominant trait. It can be inherited as a part of three distinct entities. The most common, multiple endocrine neoplasia 2A (MEN2A), is associated with pheochromocytoma and hyperparathyroidism. The second most common, MEN2B, is associated with pheochromocytoma, mucosal neuromas, and marfanoid body habitus. The least common, familial medullary thyroid cancer (FMTC), consists of medullary thyroid cancer only.

The presence of MTC has been strongly linked to the RET oncogene, located on chromosome 10. Different mutations to this gene have been demonstrated, and have variable effects on activating the RET tyrosine kinase. The discovery of this gene mutation has been studied extensively, and has had a significant effect on diagnosis, management, and our understanding of MTC. RET mutation is important to evaluate family members and consider prophylactic total thyroidectomy.

Grossly, medullary thyroid cancer is often well encapsulated. Histologically, the tumors demonstrate amyloid depositions in 60% to 80% of cases,[39] which is helpful in making the diagnosis. The tumors often display nuclear pleomorphism, necrosis, and multiple mitosis. Calcitonin staining is also helpful, and the level of staining may reflect level of cellular differentiation. Serum calcitonin levels are useful as a diagnostic and measure of response to therapy.

Medullary thyroid cancers, as a part of the APUD system, have been reported to secrete multiple polypeptide hormones besides calcitonin. Adrenocorticotropic hormone, somatostatin, vasoactive intestinal peptide, chromogranin A, neuron-specific enolase, and substance P have all been demonstrated. Carcinoembryonic antigen is also secreted by many MTCs, and has been used as a tumor marker and a receptor for nuclear imaging with octreotide imaging.

Clinically, patients tend to present with a solitary thyroid nodule, although initial presentation with a neck mass is not uncommon. Rarely, patients present with signs of local invasion, including hoarseness or dysphagia. Because of the secretory nature of these tumors, patients may present with paraneoplastic syndromes, such as Cushing or carcinoid syndrome.

Anaplastic Thyroid Cancer

Anaplastic thyroid cancer is an aggressive disease, usually proving fatal within several weeks to months of diagnosis. It represents about 3% to 5% of thyroid cancers. Pathologically, the tumor consists of grossly infiltrating tumor with areas of necrosis and hemorrhage. It often has a grey/white color and may be calcified and fibrotic. Tumors generally have high mitotic rates, marked cellular pleomorphism, necrosis, vascular invasion, and tumor emboli.[40] It may be difficult, on fine needle aspiration, to distinguish from lymphoma or other poorly differentiated thyroid cancers.

This cancer tends to affect elderly patients, and the peak incidence is in the seventh decade.[41] Several studies have shown that most patients who have this cancer have had goiter or other thyroid lesions for many years before the diagnosis of anaplastic cancer.[42] This finding leads investigators to believe that anaplastic carcinoma may represent a dedifferentiation of well-differentiated cancers.

Clinically, patients present with rapidly growing neck mass, often in the context of a slow-growing mass or goiter for several decades. Patients often present with dysphagia, dyspnea, hoarseness, sore throat, and neck pain. These are all related to the aggressive nature of the disease. Physical examination demonstrates a large, irregular neck mass, often fixed to the surrounding structures. Patients may have tracheal and esophageal involvement, and unilateral or bilateral vocal fold paralysis is not rare. Patients may demonstrate cervical metastasis. Distant metastasis tends to be to the lungs, although other sites, including bone, brain, and mediastinum, have been demonstrated.[43]

Lymphoma of the Thyroid Gland

Lymphoma of the thyroid has been reported to make up 2% to 5% of thyroid cancers. It tends to be non-Hodgkin B-cell type, although other types do occur. Patients who have a diagnosis of Hashimoto disease (chronic lymphocytic thyroiditis) have a 70-fold increased incidence of thyroid lymphoma compared with the general population.[44] It is suspected that chronic autoimmune stimulation is responsible for the development of this cancer, much the same as Sjögren disease increases the risk for lymphoma in the salivary glands.[45] Diagnosis of lymphoma in the thyroid gland requires a workup to confirm the lack of other sites of lymphoma in the body, because up to 15% of systemic lymphomas involve the thyroid gland.[46]

Many lymphomas can be diagnosed cytologically, based on their monoclonality. Differentiating them from anaplastic carcinoma is often challenging, however, and it is not uncommon to require core or open biopsy to make an accurate diagnosis.

In the clinical setting, lymphoma also mirrors anaplastic carcinoma in many ways. It tends to present with a rapidly expanding mass in the neck, often fixed to surrounding structures. Patients often have neck pain, hoarseness, dysphagia, and even facial edema. The tumor is often fixed to surrounding structures, including the trachea and larynx, the esophagus, and the skin.

Other Cancers of the Thyroid

Although rare, several other cancers can involve the thyroid, either primarily or through metastasis. Squamous cell carcinoma is a rare primary cancer of the thyroid. Once diagnosed, a thorough workup must be performed to rule out a head and neck primary that has merely metastasized to the thyroid.

Metastatic cancer to the thyroid is also rare, although well documented. It is suspected that the significant vascularity of the gland accounts for these metastases. Cancers of the kidney, lung, breast, and melanoma are the most commonly documented. In patients who have a known history of other primary cancers who have a new thyroid mass, the possibility of metastatic disease must be entertained.

EVALUATION AND MANAGEMENT OF THYROID NODULES

Thyroid nodules are common in the general population.[47] In clinical scenarios using physical examination alone, the reported incidence is about 1.5% in men and 6.4% in women.[1] In studies that included ultrasound detection, the rates vary from 19% to 67%.[48] In comparison, the incidence of thyroid cancer is rare. The lifetime risk for developing thyroid cancer is 0.73% in the United States.

(NCI SEER Cancer Statistics Review) The challenge is to distinguish between patients who are at risk for cancer and the larger percentage who have benign nodules that need no intervention.

A thorough history and physical examination are initial steps in determining risk for thyroid cancer. Several elements may help guide clinical judgment. A history of rapidly expanding neck mass, new onset of hoarseness or dysphagia, weight loss, neck or ear pain, or cough may herald a diagnosis of cancer.

Past medical history that includes neck or whole-body irradiation, exposure to radiation fallout, or growing up in iodine-deficient parts of the world may increase risk for cancer. Those who have family history of thyroid cancer, Gardner syndrome, Cowden disease, or familial polyposis also have an increased risk.

On physical examination, fixation of the mass to surrounding structures, cervical lymphadenopathy, vocal cord paralysis, or Horner syndrome should raise clinical suspicion for cancer. Age is an important factor to consider in the management of thyroid nodules. Although the incidence of nodules in children is low, the risk for cancer if a nodule is present is high, reported from 15% to 60% in the literature.[49,50] Similarly, patients older than 60 years of age also have a higher incidence of cancer in a thyroid nodule.[51] Although women have up to an eightfold higher incidence of nodules in the thyroid, the chance that a nodule is cancerous is higher in men.[52]

Some races have demonstrated a higher incidence of thyroid cancer, including Chinese, Hawaiian, and Filipino populations. The cause for this increased rate is unclear.

Laboratory Evaluation

Initial testing for patients who have a thyroid nodule should be limited to TSH level alone. A high level should prompt evaluation for hypothyroidism. A low level should prompt an evaluation for hyperthyroidism, including a free thyroxine (T4) level and a radionuclide scan to rule out a toxic adenoma of the thyroid.

Fine Needle Aspiration

Fine needle aspiration has become one of the most useful tools to help in evaluation and diagnosis of a thyroid nodule. In most series, the sensitivity and specificity are greater than 90%.[53–55] This technique has helped to significantly reduce the number of patients undergoing unnecessary thyroid surgery. There is a degree of operator dependence with the use of this technique, on the part of the clinician performing the aspiration and on the part of the cytologist reviewing the slides. In general, four outcomes may result from the needle aspiration: benign, insufficient material for diagnosis, indeterminate, or malignant. Based on these results, further evaluation or treatment may be recommended (**Fig. 4**).

Imaging of the Thyroid

The role of imaging in the preoperative evaluation of thyroid nodules has changed over time. For decades, I123- and Tc99m-labeled pertechnetate scans were the initial imaging modalities of choice for the evaluation of a thyroid nodule. Presently, these studies are considered adjunct, and ultrasound is the study of choice for evaluation of thyroid nodules. Iodine and radionuclide scanning are reserved for workup of a patient who has suspected hyperthyroidism, to rule out a toxic adenoma, or in a subset of patients who have indeterminate fine needle aspiration results, to rule out a hot nodule. The radionucleotide imaging is often still performed as a first-line diagnostic imaging study but in most cases the less expensive and less invasive ultrasound is more helpful from the standpoint of surgical decision making and determination of which patients should have cytologic sampling of the suspected mass.

Cross-sectional imaging, including CT and MR imaging, remain important in a subset of patients, especially when there is concern regarding invasion of the cancer into surrounding structures. They also prove helpful in evaluating substernal extension of tumor, and in evaluating areas not easily accessed with ultrasound, including the retropharyngeal and parapharyngeal areas. Because all of these imaging techniques are discussed in detail elsewhere in this issue, they are not addressed further here.

For surgical planning, the size of the mass, the presence of strap muscular invasion, and the presence of invasion into the esophagus and trachea are critical findings that radiologic studies can reveal. Correlating ultrasound findings with fixed anatomic landmarks, such as location relative to the cricoid, omohyoid muscle, and carotid artery, can be helpful at the time of surgery, especially in previously treated patients.

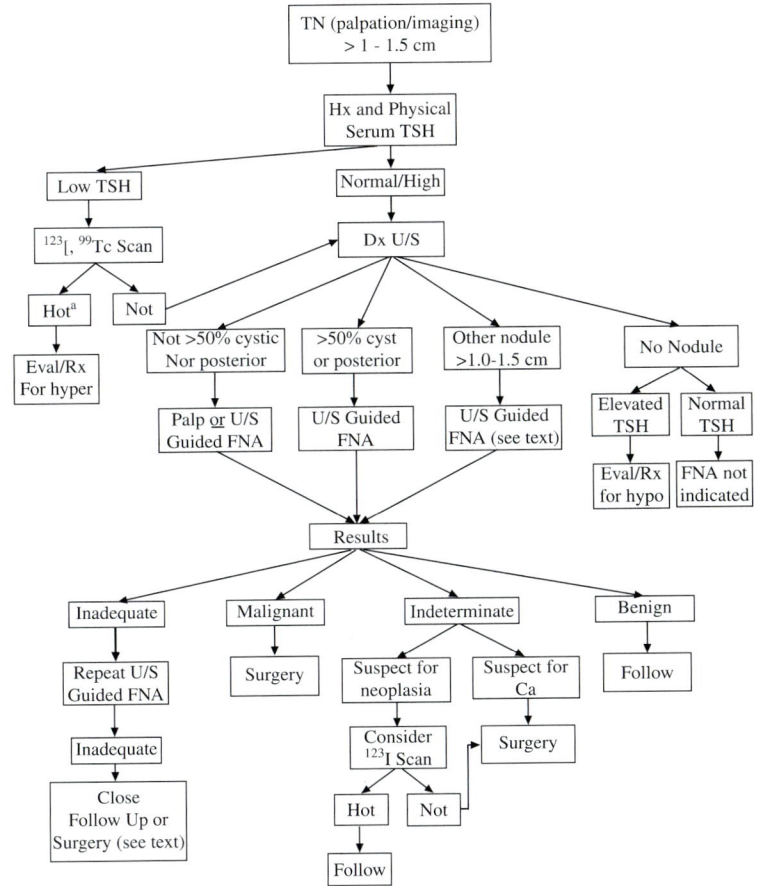

Fig. 4. Management algorithm for workup of a thyroid mass. (*From* Cooper DS, Doherty GM, Haugen BR, et al. Management guidelines for patients with thyroid nodules and differentiated thyroid cancer: the American Thyroid Association Guidelines Taskforce. Thyroid 2006;16(2):109–42. p. 112; with permission.)

THYROID SURGERY

The extent of thyroid surgery is dictated by a combination of preoperative characteristics of the thyroid tumor. Preoperative imaging of the neck and thyroid should comment, when appropriate, on any involvement of surrounding structures, extension of the thyroid into the mediastinum, obviously visible parathyroids, and pathologic or concerning adenopathy. In cases of known thyroid cancer diagnoses, attention should also be paid to the lateral neck nodes and the retropharyngeal lymph nodes, because cancers can often spread to these areas and not be visible or palpable on examination.

Unusual vascular anatomy should also be noted if visible. An anomalous retroesophageal subclavian artery is associated with a nonrecurrent laryngeal nerve on the right side of the neck, and may often be noted on preoperative imaging. Situs inversus, even rarer, is associated with a nonrecurrent laryngeal nerve on the left side of the neck. Although it is unusual, direct involvement of the vasculature in the neck or mediastinum can occur with aggressive thyroid cancers, and this knowledge is critical preoperatively. This finding often prompts vascular surgery or thoracic surgery consultation. Patients in this setting may require vascular flow studies to prepare for possible sacrifice of the carotid artery.

The pathologic type of cancer influences the extent of surgery, as does the size and extent of the tumor. Cancers with obvious extrathyroidal extension on preoperative scanning require more extensive surgery. Evidence of pathologic lymphadenopathy on imaging also affects the decision to perform central or lateral neck dissection. The operation is performed by head and neck surgeons from the fields of otolaryngology–head/neck surgery and general surgery. The procedure is performed under general anesthesia most often and through fairly small incisions in the anterior neck. The length of stay in the hospital is variable, but generally ranges from outpatient surgery to one night. The use of drainage catheters for the thyroidectomy bed is common but many surgeons are exploring not using the catheters.

Prognostic Factors and Risk Group Analysis

The prognostic factors in thyroid cancer are well described in the last 20 years. These include age, size of the tumor, distant metastases, grade of the tumor, and extrathyroidal extension. These prognostic factors are crucial. These are the same prognostic factors in different publications from Mayo Clinic, Lahey Clinic, Memorial Sloan-Kettering Cancer Center, and TNM classification.

The European Organisation for Research and Treatment of Cancer initially described these prognostic factors in 1979 and developed a scoring system.[56]

The Mayo Clinic initially described their prognostic features as AGES (age, grade of tumor, extrathyroidal extension, and size of tumor). In 1993, the Mayo Clinic updated their data and developed a new scoring system based on their prognostic features as MACIS (metastases, age, completeness of resection, invasion, and size of tumor). The major change in this scoring system was to include completeness of resection.[57] Clearly, complete surgical resection is the most important feature in the management of thyroid cancer, especially in the presence of extrathyroidal extension of the tumor.

Based on these prognostic features, Memorial Sloan-Kettering Cancer Center has divided their patients into low-, intermediate-, and high-risk groups.[5] The low-risk patients are individuals younger than the age of 45 who have low-risk tumor, whereas the high-risk patients are older than the age of 45, with high-risk features of size, histology, and extrathyroidal extension. The intermediate-risk group includes young patients who have aggressive thyroid cancers or older patients who have indolent small thyroid cancers.[58]

There continues to be a debate as to total versus less than total thyroidectomy, especially in the low-risk group patients.[16,59] There also continues to be a debate as to the extent of thyroidectomy based on size of the primary tumor. Several endocrinologists do recommend total thyroidectomy for a tumor more than 1 to 1.5 cm in size. There is no major survival difference up to 4 cm in size, however. There also seems to be considerable debate as to the indications for completion thyroidectomy in a patient who has undergone thyroid lobectomy for solitary thyroid nodule. The major emphasis here is the pathologic evaluation of the tumor and the size of the tumor. Because capsular and vascular invasion are crucial, if they are identified on final pathology report, a completion thyroidectomy is considered for facilitating radioactive iodine ablation.

Extended Thyroid Surgery

Thyroid cancer frequently spreads to the lymph nodes in the neck. Most commonly, this involves the central neck (levels VI and VII), but may also involve nodes at any level of the neck. Preoperative imaging of this region must include a comprehensive evaluation. Ultrasound is most commonly used to evaluate the lateral neck in this setting, but evaluation of the central neck and mediastinum may not be possible because of technical constraints. If evaluation of these areas becomes necessary, MR imaging or possibly CT are the modalities of choice.

Systematic evaluation of the lateral neck at the time of imaging greatly improves decision making for surgery. Concerning adenopathy may require fine needle aspiration, and definitive pathologic adenopathy requires surgical excision. Lateral neck dissection is generally reserved for the therapeutic setting (as opposed to the prophylactic setting), and surgeons often limit the extent of dissection to limit morbidity. Accurate description of the location of the nodes (by level, or by relationship to the hyoid, cricoid, carotid, and so forth) helps ensure thorough dissection of the affected areas.

Extent of Neck Dissection

There continues to be considerable debate as to the extent of neck dissection for clinically apparent metastatic nodal disease and clinically inapparent metastatic nodal disease. Our general practice is to evaluate the central compartment in all patients presenting with thyroid carcinoma. Extensive central compartment dissection is performed only if there are clinically apparent or suspicious nodes at the time of primary surgery, however.

The lateral neck dissection is reserved for patients who have clinically apparent disease, ultrasonographically proven lateral neck disease, or gross metastatic disease at the time of surgery along the jugular vein. The classic berry-picking operation has essentially been abandoned in view of high incidence of neck recurrence. Although nodal metastases have little impact on the long-term outcome in patients who have well-differentiated thyroid cancer, in older patients, especially those who have aggressive histology, there is a direct implication of neck dissection and nodal metastases, with high incidence of further recurrences. If the lateral neck nodes are clinically apparent, especially at level II, III, and IV, modified neck dissection is undertaken with extension of the thyroidectomy incision in the lateral neck. A J-shape incision or curvilinear incision may be undertaken.

The incidence of nodal metastases at level I is low, and generally level I nodes are not dissected unless there is a clinically apparent metastatic disease. The three important structures—the sternocleidomastoid muscle, the accessory nerve, and the jugular vein—are routinely preserved in thyroid neck dissection. Patients should be followed closely postoperatively with serial ultrasound and thyroglobulin to evaluate the possibility of recurrent nodal disease in the neck. Recently stimulated thyroglobulin is used in follow-up.

Laryngopharynx Surgery

Invasion of the cancer into the structures surrounding the thyroid is uncommon. The proximity of the larynx, trachea, and esophagus to the thyroid allows for cancer invasion into these areas in rare cases, however. These patients often present with clinical findings of invasion, including dysphagia, dysphonia, hemoptysis, or hematemesis. On physical examination, there may be evidence of vocal fold paralysis, tumor visible in the endolarynx and trachea, or visible invasion into the esophagus.

In some cases, patients who have invasion into the surrounding structures have few obvious findings on clinical examination. Anatomic imaging in these situations can be invaluable. Because the cancers tend to spread into the structures extrinsically, submucosal involvement is common. Accurate assessment of the extent of involvement of the underlying structures is critical; this helps prepare the patient and surgeon for possible reconstructive plans that may be needed if segments of the trachea, larynx, or esophagus are resected. CT and MR imaging are the most effective imaging techniques to evaluate for local invasiveness into the surrounding structures. Because contrast enhancement is essential for accurate evaluation in these areas, MR imaging with contrast is the study of choice in patients who are not candidates for iodine exposure because of plans for postoperative radioiodine ablation.

Surgery for Locally Advanced Thyroid Cancer

Locally advanced thyroid cancer is divided into anterior and posterior groups. Anterior extension involves the strap or sternocleidomastoid muscles. Complete resection is technically easy, with an excellent long-term outcome. When the extrathyroidal extension is noted posteriorly, however, involving the trachea, esophagus, or recurrent laryngeal nerve, the prognosis deteriorates considerably, with high incidence of local recurrence.

The principles of surgery for extrathyroidal extension remain the same as principles of oncologic surgery, which are to remove all gross tumor, preserve the vital and important structures, use adjuvant therapy, such as radioactive iodine ablation and occasionally external radiation therapy. If the tumor is involving the recurrent laryngeal nerve, and the nerve is paralyzed preoperatively, it should be sacrificed for better oncologic resection. If the nerve is functioning preoperatively, however, every effort is made to preserve the nerve. The functioning recurrent laryngeal nerve is rarely sacrificed, unless there is a high possibility of leaving gross tumor, or the tumor is encircling the nerve. These patients are routinely sent for radioactive iodine ablation.

If the tumor is adherent to the trachea, it should be divided into adherence to the tracheal wall or invasion of the trachea, with extension of the disease submucosally, or in the lumen of the trachea. If the tumor involves tracheal lumen, segmental resection of the trachea (sleeve resection) and primary anastomosis should be considered. If the tumor is only adherent to the tracheal wall, a shave procedure should be considered with satisfactory resection of all gross tumor and adjuvant therapy.

The well-differentiated thyroid cancer rarely involves the esophageal lumen, and may be adherent to the esophageal musculature, which can be easily sacrificed and resected with preservation of the continuity of the esophagus. Rarely, if the tumor is involving the esophageal lumen, esophagectomy and gastric pull up may be considered. Primary total laryngectomy is rarely indicated, unless the entire larynx is functionless or totally destroyed by the tumor. Occasionally, resection of part of the framework of the larynx or partial laryngectomy may be indicated if portion of the larynx is directly involved by the tumor.

External radiation therapy is occasionally used in patients who have high-risk thyroid cancer when gross tumor is left behind or the final histology reveals this to be poorly differentiated thyroid carcinoma. The role of external radiation therapy remains unclear in well-differentiated thyroid carcinoma. It is used in patients who have gross extrathyroidal extension to reduce the chance of local recurrence, however. It is also used for metastatic lesions, especially for the brain and the spine. The pain from bony metastasis is effectively relieved with external radiation therapy. Poorly differentiated tumors generally are not radioactive iodine avid and may be benefitted by external radiation therapy.

SUMMARY

Surgical management of thyroid carcinoma often depends on a multitude of preoperative factors. For primary treatment, radiologic evaluation often dictates the extent of surgery. For surveillance and recurrence, radiologic evaluation is the mainstay of therapy. It is therefore essential that the physicians interpreting and performing these studies be aware of the clinical and surgical correlates of their practices. This awareness not only enhances their understanding of what role these studies play in the management of their patients but also improves the patients' outcome.

REFERENCES

1. Mazzaferri EL. Management of a solitary thyroid nodule. N Engl J Med 1993;328:553–9.
2. Ezzat S, Sarti DA, Cain DR, et al. Thyroid incidentalomas. Prevalence by palpation and ultrasonography. Arch Intern Med 1994;154(16):1838–40.
3. Parkin DM, Muir CS. Cancer incidence in five continents. Comparability and quality of data. Lyon (France): IARC Scientific Publications; 1992. p. 45–173.
4. Nikiforov YE. Radiation-induced thyroid cancer: what we have learned from Chernobyl. Endocr Pathol 2006;17(4):307–17.
5. Williams ED. Chernobyl and thyroid cancer. J Surg Oncol 2006;94(8):670–7.
6. Franceschi S, Boyle P, Maisonneuve P, et al. The epidemiology of thyroid carcinoma. Crit Rev Oncog 1993;4(1):25–52.
7. Bramley MD, Harrison BJ. Papillary microcarcinoma of the thyroid gland. Br J Surg 1996;83(12):1674–83.
8. Kelemen PR, Van Herle AJ, Giuliano AE. Sentinel lymphadenectomy in thyroid malignant neoplasms. Arch Surg 1998;133(3):288–92.
9. Machens A, Holzhausen HJ, Dralle H. Skip metastases in thyroid cancer leaping the central lymph node compartment. Arch Surg 2004;139(1):43–5.
10. Mirallie E, Visset J, Sagan C, et al. Localization of cervical node metastasis of papillary thyroid carcinoma. World J Surg 1999;23(9):970–3 [discussion: 973–4].
11. Khafif A, Medina JE. Management of the neck in differentiated thyroid carcinoma. In: Randolph GW, editor. Surgery of the thyroid and parathyroid glands. Philadelphia: Elsevier Science; 2003. p. 409–18.
12. Bodenner DL, Breau RL, Suen JY. Cancer of the thyroid. In: Myers EN, Suen JY, Myers JN, editors. Cancer of the head and neck. 4th edition. Philadelphia: WB Saunders; 2003. p. 431–64.
13. Cady B, Sedgwick CE, Meissner WA, et al. Changing clinical, pathologic, therapeutic, and survival patterns in differentiated thyroid carcinoma. Ann Surg 1976;184(5):541–53.
14. Clark RL, White CE, Russel WO, et al. Clinicopathologic studies in 218 total thyroidectomies for thyroid cancer. Arq Patol 1966;38(1):25–9.
15. Carcangiu ML, Zampi G, Pupi A, et al. Papillary carcinoma of the thyroid. A clinicopathologic study of 241 cases treated at the University of Florence, Italy. Cancer 1985;55(4):805–28.
16. Mazzaferri EL, Jhiang SM. Long-term impact of initial surgical and medical therapy on papillary and follicular thyroid cancer. Am J Med 1994;

97(5):418–28 [Erratum in: Am J Med 1995 Feb;98(2):215].
17. Cady B, Rossi R. An expanded view of risk-group definition in differentiated thyroid carcinoma. Surgery 1988;104(6):947–53.
18. Crile G Jr, Antunez AR, Esselstyn CB Jr, et al. The advantages of subtotal thyroidectomy and suppression of TSH in the primary treatment of papillary carcinoma of the thyroid. Cancer 1985;55(11):2691–7.
19. Sessions R, Taylor T, Roller CA, et al. Cancer of the thyroid gland. In: Harrison LB, Sessions RB, Hong WK, editors. Head and neck cancer, a multidisciplinary approach. Philadelphia: Lippincott-Raven; 1999. p. 799–870.
20. Mazzaferri EL, Young RL, Oertel JE, et al. Papillary thyroid carcinoma: the impact of therapy in 576 patients. Medicine 1977;56(3):171–96.
21. Shaha AR. TNM classification of thyroid carcinoma. World J Surg 2007;31(5):879–87.
22. Lin JD, Chen ST, Hsueh C, et al. A 29-year retrospective review of papillary thyroid cancer in one institution. Thyroid 2007;17(6):535–41.
23. Ito Y, Miyauchi A. Lateral and mediastinal lymph node dissection in differentiated thyroid carcinoma: indications, benefits, and risks. World J Surg 2007;31(5):905–15.
24. Clark OH. Thyroid nodules and thyroid cancer: surgical aspects. West J Med 1980;133(1):1–8.
25. Harwood J, Clark OH, Dunphy JE. Significance of lymph node metastasis in differentiated thyroid cancer. Am J Surg 1978;136(1):107–12.
26. Mazzaferri EL. Papillary thyroid carcinoma: factors influencing prognosis and current therapy. Semin Oncol 1987;14(3):315–32.
27. Hoie J, Stenwig AE, Kullmann G, et al. Distant metastases in papillary thyroid cancer. A review of 91 patients. Cancer 1988;61(1):1–6.
28. Evans HL. Follicular neoplasms of the thyroid. A study of 44 cases followed for a minimum of 10 years, with emphasis on differential diagnosis. Cancer 1984;54(3):535–40.
29. Emerick GT, Duh QY, Siperstein AE, et al. Diagnosis, treatment, and outcome of follicular thyroid carcinoma. Cancer 1993;72(11):3287–95.
30. Brennan MD, Bergstralh EJ, van Heerden JA, et al. Follicular thyroid cancer treated at the Mayo Clinic, 1946 through 1970: initial manifestations, pathologic findings, therapy, and outcome. Mayo Clin Proc 1991;66(1):11–22.
31. Kahn NF, Perzin KH. Follicular carcinoma of the thyroid: an evaluation of the histologic criteria used for diagnosis. Pathol Annu 1983;18(Pt 1):221–53.
32. McDonald MP, Sanders LE, Silverman ML, et al. Hürthle cell carcinoma of the thyroid gland: prognostic factors and results of surgical treatment. Surgery 1996;120(6):1000–4.
33. Samaan NA, Schultz PN, Hickey RC, et al. The results of various modalities of treatment of well differentiated thyroid carcinomas: a retrospective review of 1599 patients. J Clin Endocrinol Metab 1992;75(3):714–20.
34. Carling T, Ocal IT, Udelsman R. Special variants of differentiated thyroid cancer: does it alter the extent of surgery versus well-differentiated thyroid cancer? World J Surg 2007;31(5):916–23.
35. Sakamoto A, Kasai N, Sugano H. Poorly differentiated carcinoma of the thyroid. A clinicopathologic entity for a high-risk group of papillary and follicular carcinomas. Cancer 1983;52(10):1849–55.
36. Flynn SD, Formann BH, Stewart AF, et al. Poorly differentiated (insular) carcinoma of the thyroid gland: an aggressive subset of differentiated thyroid neoplasms. Surgery 1988;104:963–70.
37. Killeen RM, Barnes L, Waston CG, et al. Poorly differentiated ("insular") thyroid carcinoma. Arch Otolaryngol Head Neck Surg 1990;116:1082–6.
38. Sobrinho-Simoes M, Sambade C, Fonseca E, et al. Poorly differentiated carcinomas of the thyroid gland: a review of the clinicopathologic features of a series of 28 cases of a heterogeneous, clinically aggressive group of thyroid tumors. Int J Surg Pathol 2002;10(2):123–31.
39. Papaparaskeva K, Nagel H, Droese M. Cytologic diagnosis of medullary carcinoma of the thyroid gland. Diagn Cytopathol 2000;22(6):351–8.
40. Austin JR, el-Naggar AK, Goepfert H. Thyroid cancers. II. Medullary, anaplastic, lymphoma, sarcoma, squamous cell. Otolaryngol Clin North Am 1996;29(4):611–27.
41. Trimboli P, Ulisse S, Graziano FM, et al. Trend in thyroid carcinoma size, age at diagnosis, and histology in a retrospective study of 500 cases diagnosed over 20 years. Thyroid 2006;16(11):1151–5.
42. Livolsi V, Merino M. Pathology of thyroid tumors. In: Thawley S, Panje W, Batsakis J, et al, editors. Comprehensive management of head and neck tumors. Philadelphia: WB Saunders; 1987. p. 1710–21.
43. Shvero J, Gal R, Avidor I, et al. Anaplastic thyroid carcinoma. A clinical, histologic, and immunohistochemical study. Cancer 1988;62(2):319–25.
44. Holm LE, Blomgren H, Lowhagen T. Cancer risks in patients with chronic lymphocytic thyroiditis. N Engl J Med 1985;312(10):601–4.
45. Williams ED. Malignant lymphoma of the thyroid. Clin Endocrinol Metab 1981;10(2):379–89.
46. Souhami L, Simpson WJ, Carruthers JS. Malignant lymphoma of the thyroid gland. Int J Radiat Oncol Biol Phys 1980;6(9):1143–7.
47. Rosen JE, Stone MD. Contemporary diagnostic approach to the thyroid nodule. J Surg Oncol 2006;94(8):649–61.
48. Tan GH, Gharib H. Thyroid incidentalomas: management approaches to nonpalpable nodules

discovered incidentally on thyroid imaging. Ann Intern Med 1997;126:226–31.
49. Hung W, August GP, Randolph JG, et al. Solitary thyroid nodules in children and adolescents. J Pediatr Surg 1982;17(3):225–9.
50. Kirkland RT, Kirkland JL, Rosenberg HS, et al. Solitary thyroid nodules in 30 children and report of a child with a thyroid abscess. Pediatrics 1973;51(1):85–90.
51. Pelizzo MR, Boschin IM, Toniato A, et al. Papillary thyroid carcinoma: 35-year outcome and prognostic factors in 1858 patients. Clin Nucl Med 2007;32(6):440–4.
52. Messaris G, Kyriakou K, Vasilopoulos P, et al. The single thyroid nodule and carcinoma. Br J Surg 1974;61(12):943–4.
53. Yang J, Schnadig V, Logrono R, et al. Fine-needle aspiration of thyroid nodules: A study of 4703 patients with histologic and clinical correlations. Cancer 2007;111(5):306–15.
54. Cai XJ, Valiyaparambath N, Nixon P, et al. Ultrasound-guided fine needle aspiration cytology in the diagnosis and management of thyroid nodules. Cytopathology 2006;17(5):251–6.
55. Asp AA, Georgitis W, Waldron EJ, et al. Fine needle aspiration of the thyroid. Use in an average health care facility. Am J Med 1987;83(3):489–93.
56. Shaha AR. Controversies in the management of thyroid nodule. Laryngoscope 2000;110(2 Pt 1):183–93.
57. Hay ID, Bergstralh EJ, Goellner JR, et al. Predicting outcome in papillary thyroid carcinoma: development of a reliable prognostic scoring system in a cohort of 1779 patients surgically treated at one institution during 1940 through 1989. Surgery 1993;114(6):1050–7 [discussion: 1057–8].
58. Shaha A. Treatment of thyroid cancer based on risk groups. J Surg Oncol 2006;94(8):683–91.
59. DeGroot LJ, Kaplan EL, Straus FH, et al. Does the method of management of papillary thyroid carcinoma make a difference in outcome? World J Surg 1994;18(1):123–30.

Radioiodine Imaging and Treatment in Thyroid Disorders

Wei-Shen Griggs, MD, PhD[a], Chaitanya Divgi, MD[b,c,d],*

KEYWORDS

- Thyroid • Radioiodine • Pertechnitate • Hyperthyroid
- Thyroiditis • Goiter • Differentiated thyroid cancer
- Imaging • Gamma camera

The thyroid is one of the largest endocrine glands. It produces thyroid hormones that regulate metabolism and are essential to proper development and differentiation of the cells in the body. Iodine is an essential element in thyroid hormone synthesis. The thyroid has the ability to concentrate and incorporate iodine into thyroid hormone. Incorporation of iodine is essential to the formation of thyroid hormone.

Radioactive iodine is one of the first radioisotopes to be used in medicine. Radioactive iodine is taken up and incorporated in an identical manner as nonradioactive iodine by the thyroid gland. It has been used to evaluate and treat benign and malignant thyroid diseases for more than 50 years.

The following discussions refer to the patient population in the United States.

INSTRUMENTATION

Most radioiodine imaging is currently performed using a gamma camera. The most commonly used radioactive isotopes of iodine are iodine-123 (I-123), which emits only gamma rays (also called photons) with an energy of 159 KeV, and iodine-131 (I-131), which has a complex decay scheme that includes photons of 364 KeV. Radioactive iodine is usually administered orally. It accumulates in the thyroid and is best visualized 4 hours or more after administration. Photons emitted from the thyroid enter the gamma camera and interact with the crystal to produce scintillations that are detected, amplified, and converted into light. An image of radioactive iodine distribution is thus created. Modern cameras have designs that are digital, with improved efficiency in photon capture. Because the photon energies of I-123 and I-131 are different, they require different collimators—low energy collimation for I-123 and high energy for I-131.

Fig. 1 illustrates the basic principles of a gamma camera.

PATIENT PREPARATION

All patients presenting for radioiodine imaging or therapy should discontinue use of iodine-containing supplements or medications that can potentially affect the ability of iodine uptake and incorporation by the thyroid gland.[1] Most centers also recommend a low iodine diet for 7 to 14 days before radioiodine.

For patients who have thyroid cancer, the optimal condition for imaging and treatment is elevation of serum thyrotropin (TSH) level. This elevation can be achieved endogenously by withdrawing thyroid hormone and waiting until

---

[a] Fairfax Radiological Consultants, PC, 2722 Merrilee Drive, Suite 203, Fairfax, VA 22031, USA
[b] Wistar Institute, Philadelphia, PA 19104, USA
[c] Abramson Cancer Center, University of Pennsylvania, Philadelphia, PA 19104, USA
[d] Nuclear Medicine and Clinical Molecular Imaging, Hospital of the University of Pennsylvania, 3400 Spruce Street - Donner 116, Philadelphia, PA 19104, USA
* Corresponding author. Nuclear Medicine and Clinical Molecular Imaging, Hospital of the University of Pennsylvania, 3400 Spruce Street - Donner 116, Philadelphia, PA 19104.
E-mail address: chaitanya.divgi@uphs.upenn.edu (C. Divgi).

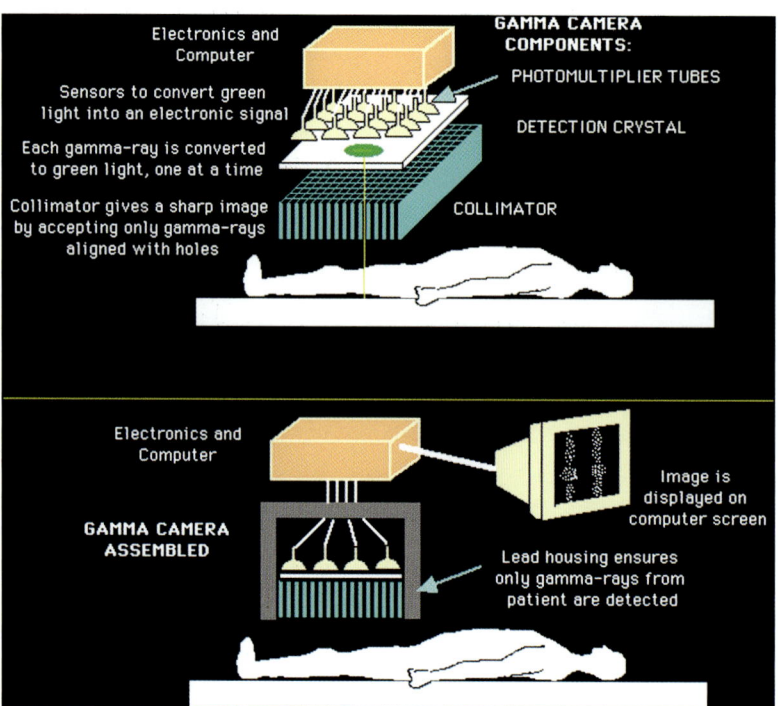

Fig. 1. A gamma (Anger) camera. (*Courtesy of* Douglas J. Wagenaar, PhD, Northridge, CA. Available at: http://www.med.harvard.edu/JPNM/physics/didactics/basics.html.)

the serum TSH is 30 mIU/L or greater. Elevation of TSH can also be achieved exogenously by administration of recombinant human TSH (rhTSH), given intramuscularly 0.9 mg on two consecutive days. It is indicated in patients who cannot be prepared by total thyroidectomy, or in the presence of sufficient functioning tumor, or with pituitary insufficiency, or in patients who cannot tolerate prolonged hypothyroidism. The recent FDA approval of rhTSH for the diagnosis and treatment of patients who have thyroid cancer has increased its use, although the cost is high. It is also increasingly used routinely for follow-up imaging in low-risk patients.

For diagnostic purposes, radioactivity is given to women of childbearing age only if the patient reports not being pregnant. Therapeutic radioactivity is given to women of childbearing age within 48 hours of a negative serum β-HCG test. Pregnancy status does not need to be checked if the woman is postmenopausal (defined by convention as no menstrual period for at least a year), or the woman has been rendered incapable of childbearing surgically or medically. Following radioiodine therapy, women should not become pregnant until the medical condition has been optimized. Some centers suggest a waiting period of 6 months and 12 months for hyperthyroidism and thyroid cancer, respectively, after radioiodine treatment. Because iodide is also a component of milk, lactating women undergoing radioiodine therapy should be asked to stop breastfeeding until accumulation in the breasts is minimal. Therapy should be delayed whenever possible until lactation ends, failing which frequent expression of milk is recommended to minimize radiation to the breasts.

Elderly or cardiac patients who have Graves disease may require antithyroid medications before radioactive iodine treatment so as to minimize the risk for excessive hormone release due to radiation thyroiditis.

ISOTOPES

The most common radioactive iodine isotopes in clinical use today are I-123 and I-131. I-123 is produced in a cyclotron and decays by electron capture with a half-life of 13.6 hours. It emits gamma ray photons at 159 keV. I-131 is produced in a generator and has a half-life of 8.05 days. It emits 364 keV photons and beta particles with an average energy of 192 keV. I-131 can thus be used for both imaging and therapy. I-123 has better imaging characteristics for gamma camera imaging; however it is more expensive.

Tc-99m pertechnetate is also trapped by thyroid follicular cells and can be used for thyroid scintigraphic imaging. Unlike radioactive iodine, Tc-99m pertechnetate is not incorporated into thyroid hormone. It is therefore not used for functional evaluation of the thyroid. In rare situations, a hypofunctioning nodule on radioactive iodine imaging may have normal uptake of Tc-99m pertechnetate, creating a "discordant nodule."

Table 1 summarizes the salient physical and radiation absorbed dose characteristics of the commonly used isotopes.[2] The radiation absorbed dose to patients varies depending on thyroid uptake.[3]

I-124 is a positron emitter. It emits positrons in approximately 23% of decays, with an average energy of 819 keV. It has a half-life of 4.18 days. Imaging of thyroid disorder with I-124 positron emission tomography (PET) is still experimental but seems extremely promising. Its cost is also currently high, precluding routine use.

IMAGING AND TREATMENT OF BENIGN THYROID DISORDERS

Thyroid nodules, signs and symptoms of hyper- or hypothyroidism, are the most common benign thyroid disorders evaluated using nuclear medicine techniques.

A sensitive serum TSH assay is an integral part of such evaluation, being the most sensitive test for confirming clinically apparent and mild subclinical thyroid hormone excess or deficiency. This test is usually a component of thyroid function tests, which typically include serum thyroxine (T4) measurements. Most thyroxine is protein-bound. Other laboratory tests may include free T4 and triiodothyronine (T3) and free T3, especially if the patient is clinically hyperthyroid and has low/undetectable serum TSH. Thyroid autoantibodies, such as TSH receptor antibodies, thyroid-stimulating immunoglobulins, and antithyroperoxidase, are also sometimes obtained to determine possible autoimmune causes for thyroid disorders.

Radioiodine imaging for benign thyroid disorders is performed with 0.2 to 0.5 mCi I-123 or 0.02 to 0.05 mCi I-131. Some nuclear medicine physicians use 2 to 5 mCi Tc-99m pertechnetate for imaging the thyroid, whereas thyroid radioiodine uptake is measured with I-123 or I-131.

Diffuse Goiter

Hyperthyroid

Graves disease The most common cause for hyperthyroidism is Graves disease, also called toxic diffuse goiter. Autoantibodies against TSH receptors on cells of thyroid develop in patients who have Graves disease, thereby stimulating the thyroid cells and increasing thyroid hormone production. The patients usually have symptoms associated with hyperthyroidism and some patients may also develop thyroid ophthalmopathy. Laboratory abnormalities include suppressed TSH and elevated T3 and T4. As seen in **Fig. 2**, radioiodine imaging shows a diffusely enlarged thyroid gland with increased uptake. A pyramidal lobe can also be seen sometimes. Some patients may have a normal-sized gland with increased uptake.

I-131 is the treatment of choice for Graves disease. Physicians usually prefer to treat the patients with I-131 with a dose to render the patients hypothyroid, because calculation of a dose that would result in a euthyroid state is difficult; treatment effects can be prolonged, with a variable time to euthyroid or hypothyroid state, and it is easier to treat hypothyroidism than hyperthyroidism. The patients subsequently require thyroid hormone replacement for life.

Subacute and silent thyroiditis Patients who have subacute or silent thyroiditis can present with diffuse goiter and thyrotoxicosis during the inflammatory phase. They are distinguished from Graves disease by decreased radioactive iodine uptake and minimal thyroid activity on radioiodine imaging (**Fig. 3**). The thyrotoxicosis results from release of stored thyroid hormone secondary to infiltration and disruption of the thyroid follicles by the giant cells in subacute thyroiditis and lymphocytes in silent thyroiditis. These two disorders can be further distinguished by their different clinical presentation. Patients who have subacute thyroiditis often present with neck pain and report a history of preceding viral (usually upper respiratory) infection. Patients who have silent thyroiditis usually do not

Table 1				
Physical and radiation–absorbed dose characteristics of the commonly used isotopes				
Radionuclide	Half-life	Primary Photon (KeV)	Beta Energy (Average)	Radiation Absorbed Dose (cGy/µCi)
Tc-99m	6 h	140	None	0.0002
I-123	13 h	159	None	0.013
I-131	8 d	364	192 KeV	0.13

Data from Rosenberg RD, Mettler FA Jr, Moseley RD Jr, et al. Thyroid radiation absorbed dose from diagnostic procedures in U.S. population. Radiology 1985;156:183–5.

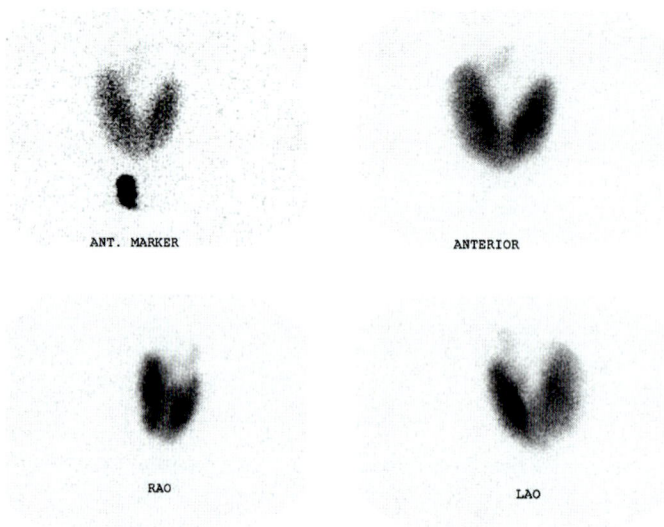

Fig. 2. Anterior with and without marker at sternal notch, left anterior oblique and right anterior oblique views of the thyroid in a patient who had Graves disease. There is diffusely increased uptake by the thyroid gland, with 2-hour and 24-hour uptake of 92% and 98%, respectively. A pyramidal lobe can be faintly seen arising from the superior aspect of the right lobe.

have gland tenderness. Postpartum thyroiditis is a subtype of silent thyroiditis in the postpartum period.

Subacute thyroiditis is treated with nonsteroidal anti-inflammatory drugs and steroids in more severe cases. Silent thyroiditis is a self-limiting disorder that usually does not require treatment.

Hypothyroid

Chronic thyroiditis Chronic thyroiditis is a common cause of hypothyroidism. The most common cause of primary hypothyroidism is chronic autoimmune thyroiditis, or Hashimoto thyroiditis. Hashimoto thyroiditis has a wide range of clinical presentations, laboratory results, and imaging findings. The symptoms are related to duration and severity of hypothyroidism, the time course of development of hypothyroidism, and psychologic characteristics of the patient.[4] The thyroid may be enlarged, atrophic, or normal size, and it may contain nodules. The nodules may infrequently harbor thyroid cancer or lymphoma. Laboratory tests, sometimes discordant, may reveal increased TSH and decreased free T4 in overt or clinical hypothyroidism, or increased TSH and normal free T4 and T3 in subclinical hypothyroidism. Thyroid autoantibodies are positive in 95% of patients who have Hashimoto thyroiditis.

Clinical hypothyroidism is treated with levothyroxine replacement. Treatment of subclinical hypothyroidism with levothyroxine is controversial.

Subacute and silent thyroiditis Subacute and silent thyroiditis often follow a triphasic course. They have a period of hypothyroidism following initial stage of thyrotoxicosis, which is then followed by recovery to euthyroid state. During the period of hypothyroidism, there is often discordance between the laboratory values and clinical status. Radioiodine thyroid uptake usually remains minimal and there is minimal thyroid activity on radioiodine imaging. During the recovery phase, however, there may be diffusely increased uptake that may mimic Graves disease.[5] In thyroiditis, this period is transient and is followed by returning to baseline. Repeat imaging and discordant laboratory values help make this distinction.

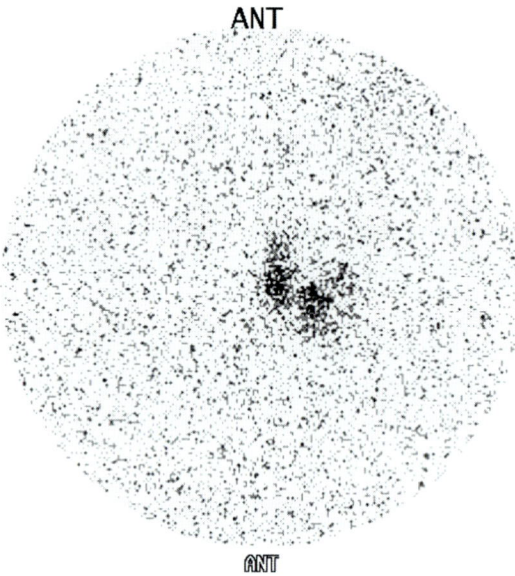

Fig. 3. Anterior view of the thyroid in a patient who had biopsy-proven lymphocytic thyroiditis. There is markedly decreased uptake by the thyroid with relative high background on this image obtained with parallel hole because of low uptake. Neck uptake (24 hour) is 1.6%.

Nodule Evaluation

Thyroid nodules are common. It is estimated that about 4% to 7% of the United States population aged 50 years and older have clinically apparent thyroid nodules.[6] More than 50% of thyroids have nodules when examined on ultrasound.[7] Thyroid nodules may be solitary or multiple. On ultrasound, the nodules may be cystic or solid or mixed cystic and solid. A thyroid with a single palpable nodule on clinical examination may contain multiple nodules on ultrasound or other imaging modalities.

A multinodular goiter is a clinical diagnosis made on physical examination. Multinodular goiter is found to be more prevalent in endemic areas, believed to be related to goitrogenic substance intake or iodine deficiency.

Most thyroid nodules are benign. About 5% of thyroid nodules are malignant. The risk for cancer is probably not significantly different between solitary nodule and multinodular goiter. The primary purpose of evaluation of the thyroid nodules is to exclude malignant lesions. Although ultrasound remains the mainstay of thyroid nodule evaluation, thyroid scintigraphy can be used in special situations to aid the evaluation.

According to the American Association of Clinical Endocrinologists and Association Medici Endocrinologi Medical Guidelines for Clinical Practice for the Diagnosis and Management of Thyroid Nodules, thyroid scintigraphy is indicated for the following:

- Single thyroid nodule or multinodular goiter (MNG) and suppressed serum TSH
- Large MNG, especially with substernal extension
- In search of ectopic thyroid tissue (for example, struma ovarii or sublingual thyroid)
- In subclinical hyperthyroidism to identify occult hyperfunctioning tissue
- Some investigators suggest evaluation of follicular neoplasms with a scintiscan to identify a functioning cellular adenoma that may be benign; however, most such nodules are cold on a scintiscan. On thyroid scintigraphy, nodules can be hyperfunctioning (ie, "hot") or can be hypofunctioning (ie, "cold"). Hot nodules are almost always benign. There is a 5% to 8% risk for malignancy in cold nodules

Solitary nodule

Hyperfunctioning nodule A solitary hyperfunctioning nodule is frequently caused by hyperfunctioning thyroid adenoma. The risk for thyrotoxicity is increased with nodule size. Most hyperfunctioning nodules are autonomous (not under the regulation of TSH). An autonomously hyperfunctioning nodule can suppress iodine uptake by the rest of the gland, as seen in an example in **Fig. 4**.

I-131 is the preferred therapy for thyrotoxicosis attributable to a hyperfunctioning nodule because a large portion of the administered radioactivity is concentrated in the hyperfunctioning nodule. Often, return of function to the normal tissue can be expected afterward. If there is a nodule that

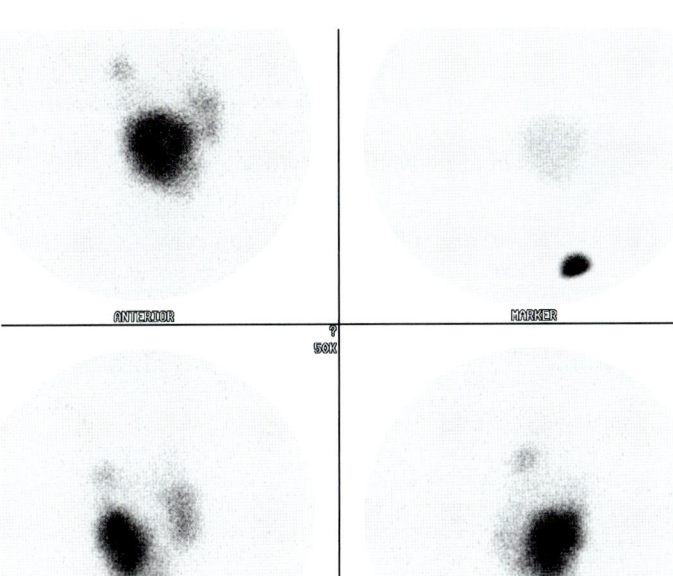

Fig. 4. Anterior with and without marker at sternal notch, left anterior oblique and right anterior oblique views of the thyroid in a patient who had hyperthyroid symptoms. There is a dominant functioning nodule with suppression of the rest of the gland. Neck uptake at 2 hours and 24 hours is 9% and 42%, respectively.

causes compressive symptoms, surgery may be necessary.

Hypofunctioning nodule Because there is a 5% to 8% risk for malignancy in the cold nodules, fine needle aspiration is generally recommended for further evaluation, unless the nodule is shown by ultrasound to be entirely cystic.

Multinodular goiter
Hyperthyroid Some of the nodules in a multinodular goiter may develop to become autonomously functioning nodules. The autonomously functioning nodule may secrete enough thyroid hormone and render the patient hyperthyroid. This nodule may suppress iodine uptake by the rest of the thyroid. On laboratory testing, TSH is often suppressed and thyroid hormone is often mildly elevated. Thyroid scintigraphy shows heterogeneous uptake within the gland, with hot and cold nodules. There is normal or elevated radioactive iodine uptake. **Fig. 5** is an example of a toxic multinodular goiter.

After ultrasound evaluation and, when indicated, a fine needle aspiration that rules out malignancy, toxic multinodular goiter is most frequently treated with I-131. Surgery to remove the gland may be necessary if there are symptoms of compression by the goitrous thyroid.

Euthyroid I-131 is sometimes used to reduce goiter size to alleviate mass effect, especially in patients who choose not to undergo surgery or in whom surgery is contraindicated. The dose of I-131 in these patients is significantly higher than that for Graves disease or a toxic multinodular goiter. The efficacy of such therapy is variable.

Hypothyroid This condition can be seen in thyroiditis, as discussed earlier.

IMAGING, TREATMENT, AND FOLLOW-UP OF DIFFERENTIATED THYROID CANCER
General

Thyroid cancer, staging, and risk assessment
Although thyroid cancer is the most common endocrine malignancy, clinically recognized thyroid cancer composes less than 1% of all human malignancies. Thyroid cancer is two to three times more frequent in females than males. It is the eighth most common malignancy in females.[8] The preferred management strategy for differentiated thyroid cancer is still under debate, because of a lack of carefully controlled prospective clinical trials. A well-designed trial for differentiated thyroid cancer is of course difficult because of the low incidence, prolonged course, and natural history of the disease.

About 80% of thyroid cancers are of follicular cell origin, and are of papillary, follicular, Hürthle cell, or anaplastic types. Papillary thyroid cancer is the most common subtype. Differentiated thyroid cancers are composed of papillary and follicular thyroid cancers. As follicular thyroid cancer can have a variable amount of Hürthle cells, Hürthle cell cancer is considered by some to be a variant of follicular cancer or there is a spectrum between follicular and Hürthle cell cancers.

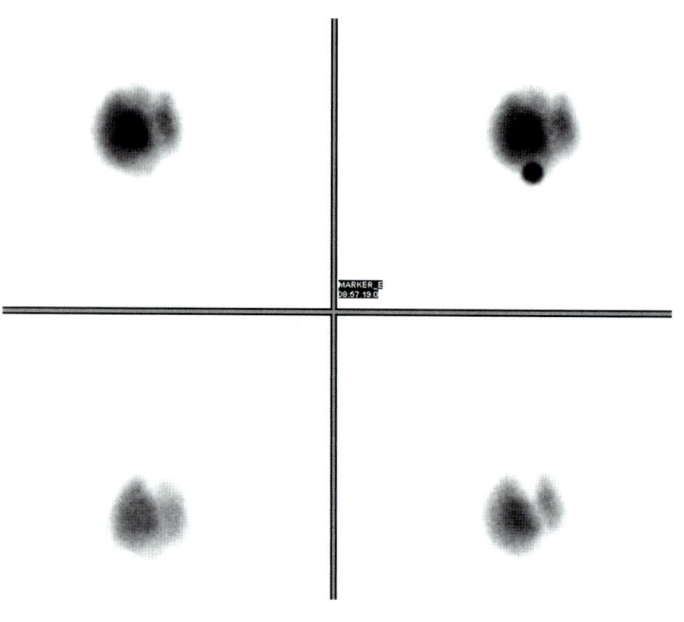

Fig. 5. Hyperthyroid multinodular goiter. The increased uptake in several nodules, with absence of uptake in the remainder of the gland, is evident.

Hürthle cell cancer is thus considered by some to be a differentiated thyroid cancer. I-131 is used in the treatment of differentiated thyroid cancers that accumulate iodine, and has no role in the treatment of undifferentiated carcinomas unless they contain thyroid follicular elements that can concentrate radioiodine.

The prognosis of differentiated thyroid cancer is related to patient and tumor factors. The patient factors include patient age, gender, and family history. The tumor factors include tumor histologic grade, size of tumor, extrathyroidal extension, and distant metastasis. The importance of local lymph node metastasis on prognosis is controversial; it is becoming increasingly accepted that nodal metastases impact recurrence-free, but not overall, survival. The most recent guidelines for the management of differentiated thyroid cancer stress that age is the most important determinant of risk.[9]

Patients who have thyroid cancer can be divided into low-, intermediate-, and high-risk groups based on these factors. An excellent comparison of the various staging systems used in prognosis of patients who have thyroid cancer can be found in the review by Lang and colleagues.[10]

Radioiodine imaging and treatment of differentiated thyroid cancer

Surgical resection of the primary tumor is the preferred initial treatment of thyroid cancer. Extent of surgery and the necessity for lymph node dissection and subsequent management have been standardized.[9] Near-total or total thyroidectomy is the preferred operation in most patients, because there is a high prevalence of thyroid cancer in the contralateral lobe and postoperative I-131 treatment is more effective after total thyroidectomy. According to National Comprehensive Cancer Network Guidelines, total lobectomy alone can be performed in a patient with no risk factors and who does not have a history of neck radiation exposure, and has either a less than 1-cm papillary tumor that is unifocal and confined to thyroid without vascular invasion or a less than 4-cm follicular cancer without or with minimal invasion. Completion thyroidectomy is recommended for patients who have had lobectomy for tumors larger than T1 (>1 cm) or locally invasive cancer or have metastasis, recurrent cancer, or tumor in the resection margin.[11]

Many patients who have had near-total or total thyroidectomy have thyroid remnants identifiable on radioiodine imaging. Although there is still debate about the necessity of I-131 treatment of thyroid remnant after total thyroidectomy, many clinicians prefer to treat residual thyroid tissue with I-131 (ablation). There is decreased recurrence and disease-specific mortality when postoperative I-131 treatment is used as part of initial treatment, especially in high-risk patients.[12–14] I-131 thyroid remnant ablation seeks to achieve elimination of any functioning thyroid tissue to facilitate follow-up with thyroglobulin measurements and radioiodine imaging and any potential microscopic cancer in the thyroid bed or micrometastasis. A large thyroid remnant also acts to suppress the TSH, which is necessary for tumor uptake of I-131.[11] Posttreatment imaging is frequently performed to confirm targeting of I-131 to tissue of thyroid origin and to detect additional residual tumor/tissue or metastasis. Treating a large thyroid remnant with I-131 is complicated by the risk for radiation thyroiditis and possibly thyrotoxicosis. A completion thyroidectomy is frequently performed after lobectomy if I-131 treatment is deemed necessary.

The amount of diagnostic radioiodine used is under dispute; most groups recommend the lowest possible amount required before I-131 treatment because of concern for "stunning" (decrease of therapeutic radioiodine uptake by remnant thyroid tissue or metastasis after administration of a diagnostic I-131 dose). Stunning is a radiobiologic phenomenon caused by radiation damage from the imaging dose of I-131, rather than a transient inability of thyroid remnant or differentiated thyroid cancer to take up radioactive iodine.[15] Most institutions use less than 5 mCi I-131 for diagnostic purposes to avoid stunning. In our institution, I-123 is preferred for its better imaging characteristics; its favorable radiation absorbed dose also obviates stunning at the amounts used.

There are three approaches to choosing a dose of I-131 for treatment: a fixed amount of I-131,[16] quantitative tumor dosimetry,[17] and treatment with the maximum tolerated dose, using upper limits set based on blood and whole-body radiation absorbed dose.[18] There has been no prospective randomized trial to determine which is better. Several analyses and studies have suggested that these approaches yield similar results, however, and as a consequence a fixed dose in the range of 75 to 200 mCi is favored.[19–23] At our center, a dose of I-131 is selected based on risk assessment, pathology results, and diagnostic radioiodine imaging findings.

After I-131 treatment, patients are treated with levothyroxine. The amount of levothyroxine is generally selected to provide a euthyroid state and to suppress TSH secretion. Overt hyperthyroidism caused by excess thyroid hormone should be avoided.

All patients presenting for radioactive iodine imaging and treatment should follow the preparation as described above.

Follow-up of differentiated thyroid cancer

Long-term surveillance is necessary because long-term survival is common and the patients are at risk for tumor recurrence or metastasis. Follow-up of differentiated thyroid cancer involves a combination of physical examination, laboratory testing, and imaging.

Laboratory testing includes measurement of serum thyroglobulin, TSH, and T4. Thyroid tissue is the only source of circulating thyroglobulin, and thus serum thyroglobulin should be undetectable after total or near-total thyroidectomy and successful I-131 treatment. Serum thyroglobulin is a particularly useful and specific tumor marker for differentiated thyroid cancer, after total or near-total thyroidectomy and I-131 treatment. Serum thyroglobulin can be measured without TSH stimulation, or under TSH stimulation. TSH stimulation is achieved either through thyroid hormone withdrawal and maintenance on a low-iodine diet, or, more commonly, through administration of recombinant TSH. Antithyroglobulin antibody is usually measured in conjunction with serum thyroglobulin. The measurement of serum thyroglobulin is unreliable when antithyroglobulin antibody is present. It has been suggested that serum thyroglobulin level does not increase as much with rhTSH stimulation as with thyroid hormone withdrawal,[23] although rhTSH is used increasingly, primarily for patient convenience—hypothyroidism is uncomfortable for most patients.[24]

Imaging methods include radioiodine whole-body imaging and anatomic imaging of the neck with ultrasound or MR imaging. Chest radiograph is no longer used for routine follow-up. A whole-body radioiodine scan is performed with 1 to 10 mCi I-123 or up to 5 mCi I-131 (stunning is less of a concern in the follow-up period). Radioiodine whole-body imaging can be performed after thyroid hormone withdrawal or rhTSH stimulation. There is some concern that faster iodide clearance in the euthyroid, TSH-stimulated state can decrease sensitivity of radioiodine imaging in this setting;[25] at least one study has shown that stimulation by thyroid hormone withdrawal or rhTSH injection did not produce a statistically significant difference in whole-body I-131 imaging findings when a minimum of 4 mCi of I-131 was used.[23] Most groups prefer to carry out follow-up studies with I-131.

Low-Risk Patients

These patients have excellent long-term survival. Thyroid lobectomy versus total thyroidectomy may not produce differences in long-term survival, but there are reports that total thyroidectomy is associated with increased disease-free survival.[26,27] Most clinicians now opt for total or near-total thyroidectomy, in keeping with recent guidelines.[9]

I-131 thyroid remnant treatment in these patients is also controversial.[9] If the patient receives I-131 treatment, monitoring consists of initial evaluation at the time of remnant treatment and subsequent follow-up. If patients have low-risk differentiated thyroid cancer with no evidence of disease at 6- and 12-month follow-up and serum thyroglobulin and antithyroglobulin are negative, diagnostic whole-body radioactive iodine scan adds no information and thus may not be indicated.[28-30]

Intermediate- and High-Risk Patients

Initial presentation

The extent of initial surgical treatment or whether to have completion thyroidectomy is under debate for patients who have intermediate-risk disease, although increasingly this population is treated similarly to those who have high-risk disease (ie, total thyroidectomy, with neck dissection when appropriate).[9,11] Patients who have intermediate-risk differentiated thyroid cancer may have had a lobectomy and present for residual thyroid lobe treatment, or more likely, have had near-total or total thyroidectomy and present for thyroid remnant treatment.

If debulking of the tumor is not possible or cannot be performed, it is considered unresectable. This situation is rare and is not discussed here.

Up to 10% of children who have differentiated thyroid cancer present with synchronous metastases, especially in the lung.[31] About 4% to 6% of patients who have high-risk thyroid cancer present with synchronous metastases.[32-34] Some patients may initially present with pathologic fractures secondary to bone metastasis from differentiated thyroid cancer. Differentiated thyroid cancer can over time metastasize to distant lymph nodes, lungs, bone, other solid organs, and the central nervous system. In general, diffuse lung metastasis with a micronodular pattern or normal chest radiograph or chest CT have better response to radioactive iodine treatment than macronodular pattern.[34] Metastasis to bone, liver, and brain are difficult to treat.

Follow-up after initial treatment

Patients are initially followed up with TSH-stimulated thyroglobulin measurement at regular intervals supplemented with imaging, including radioactive iodine whole-body scan and anatomic

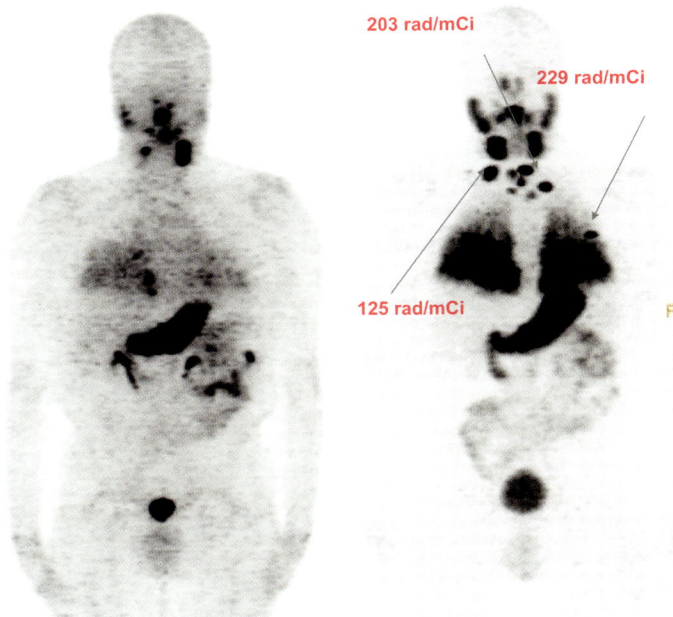

Fig. 6. Iodine-124 whole-body PET image (*left*) and calculated radiation absorbed doses to lesions (*right*) in a patient who had thyroid cancer metastatic to lungs and lymph nodes.

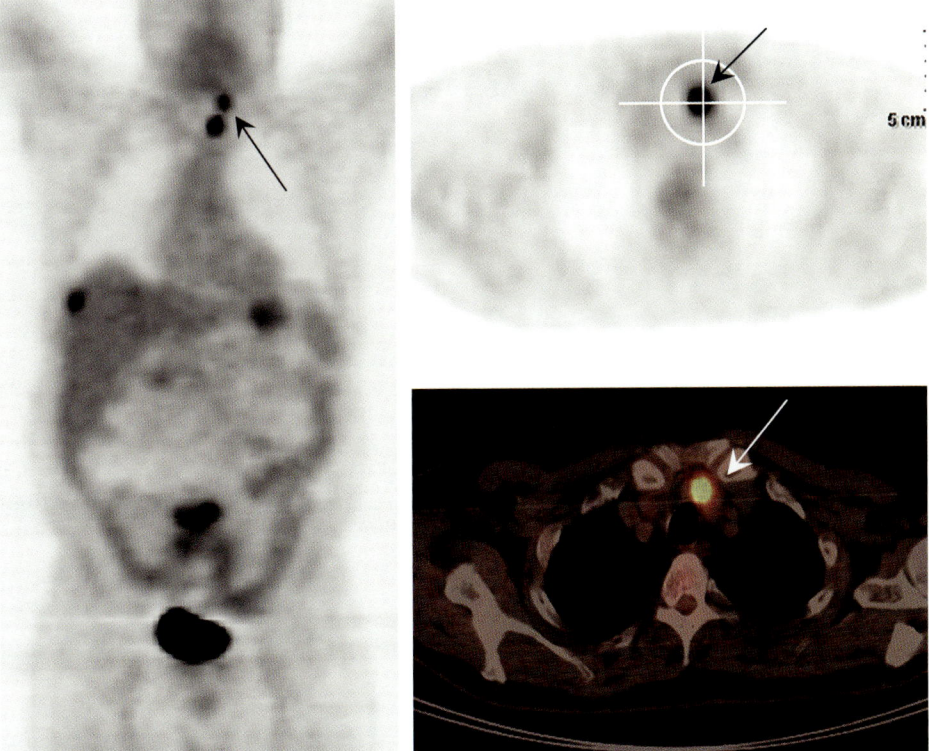

Fig. 7. A patient who had colon carcinoma metastatic to the liver had an FDG PET for extent of disease evaluation. A thyroid focus (*arrow*) was found to be papillary carcinoma. A maximum intensity projection whole-body image (*left*), a transaxial PET image through the thyroid (*center*), and a "fused" image of the PET and CT (*right*) are displayed.

imaging, either ultrasound or MR imaging of the neck. The patient is considered free of disease after one or two negative radioiodine whole-body imaging scans and without increase in thyroglobulin. Patients free of disease may be followed with annual non–TSH-stimulated thyroglobulin measurement.[9]

High-risk disease frequently becomes non–iodine avid. Preliminary results indicate that I-124 PET imaging may be more sensitive than I-131 whole-body planar imaging for detecting recurrent tumor or metastasis.[35]

Non–iodine avid disease These patients are followed with TSH-stimulated thyroglobulin. They can still be treated with I-131 and 16% to 18% of these patients demonstrate positive results on post I-131 treatment scan.[34,36] Patients who have negative I-131 (or I-123) diagnostic scans may benefit from stimulated I-124 PET scans. **Fig. 6** demonstrates a whole-body I-124 image in a patient; serial quantitative imaging permitted calculation of tumor radiation absorbed dose.

Patients who have negative I-131 posttreatment scans are considered to have non–iodine avid disease[37] and are candidates for experimental therapeutics with targeting agents, including kinase inhibitors.[38] These may not only elicit tumor response but also promote tumor redifferentiation with return of iodine avidity.

THYROID INCIDENTALOMAS

The increasing use of whole-body PET imaging, using [18F]-fluorodeoxyglucose (FDG), has increased the incidence of incidentally identified thyroid nodules.[7,39] **Fig. 7** is an example of a patient who had metastatic colon carcinoma in whom a thyroid nodule (papillary cancer at biopsy) was discovered in an FDG PET scan performed for extent of disease evaluation. Diffuse thyroid FDG uptake is generally benign, whereas focal lesions tend to have a higher probability of being malignant.

SUMMARY

Thyroid disorders may be imaged and treated with radioiodine. Iodine uptake by thyroid follicular cells lends itself to imaging of functional characteristics of the gland. Gamma camera and, increasingly, PET imaging of thyroid disorders permit delineation of thyroid functional status. Iodine uptake also permits treatment, using I-131, of hyperthyroid disease and cancer, for which I-131 is the primary treatment.

REFERENCES

1. Meiner DA, Brill DR, Becker DV, et al. Procedure guideline for therapy of thyroid disease with 131 iodine. J Nucl Med 2002;43(6):856–61.
2. Rosenberg RD, Mettler FA Jr, Moseley RD Jr, et al. Thyroid radiation absorbed dose from diagnostic procedures in U.S. population. Radiology 1985;156:183–5.
3. Stabin MG, Watson EE, Marcus CD, et al. Radiation dosimetry for adult female and fetus from I-131 administration in hyperthyroidism. J Nucl Med 1991;32:808–13.
4. AACE Thyroid Task Force. American Association of Clinical Endocrinologists medical guidelines for clinical practice for the evaluation and treatment of hyperthyroidism and hypothyroidism. Endocr Pract 2002;8(6):457–69.
5. Intenzo CM, dePapp AE, Fabbour S, et al. Scintigraphic manifestations of thyrotoxicosis. Radiographics 2003;23:857–69.
6. Mazzaferri EL. Management of a solitary thyroid nodule. N Engl J Med 1993;328:553–9.
7. Ezzat S, Sarti DA, Cain DR, et al. Thyroid incidentalomas: prevalence by palpation and ultrasonography. Arch Intern Med 1994;154:1838–40.
8. Ries LAG, Melbert D, Krapcho M, et al, editors. SEER cancer statistics review, 1975–2004. Bethesda: National Cancer Institute; 2007. Available at: http://seer.cancer.gov/csr/1975_2004/. Accessed May 8, 2008.
9. Cooper DS, Doherty GM, Haugen BR, et al. Management guidelines for patients with thyroid nodules and differentiated thyroid cancer. Thyroid 2006;16:109–42.
10. Lang BH-H, Lo C-Y, Chan W-F, et al. Staging systems for papillary thyroid carcinoma: a review and comparison. Ann Surg 2007;245:366–78.
11. Mazzaferri EL, Kloos RT. Current approaches to primary therapy for papillary and follicular thyroid caner. J Clin Endocrinol Metab 2001;86(4):1447–63.
12. Mazzaferri EL, Jhiang SM. Long-term impact of initial surgical and medical therapy on papillary and follicular thyroid cancer. Am J Med 1994;97:418–28.
13. DeGroot LJ, Kaplan EL, Straus FH, et al. Does the method of management of papillary thyroid carcinoma make a difference in outcome? World J Surg 1994;18:123–30.
14. Taylor T, Specker B, Robbins J, et al. Outcome after treatment of high-risk papillary and non-Hürthle-cell follicular thyroid carcinoma. Ann Intern Med 1998;129:622–7.
15. Yeung WD, Humm JL, Larson SM. Radioiodine uptake in thyroid remnants during therapy after tracer dosimetry. J Nucl Med 2000;41(6):1082–5.
16. Beirwaltes WH, Rabbani R, Dmuchowski C, et al. An analysis of "ablation of thyroid remnants" with I-131 in 511 patients from 1947–1984: experience at University of Michigan. J Nucl Med 1984;25(12):1287–91.

17. Maxon HR, Englaro EE, Thomas SR, et al. Radioiodine-131 therapy for well-differentiated thyroid cancer—a quantitative radiation dosimetric approach: outcome and validation in 85 patients. J Nucl Med 1992;33:1132–6.
18. Benua RS, Cicale NR, Sonenberg M, et al. The relation of radioiodine dosimetry to results and complications in the treatment of metastatic thyroid cancer. AJR Am J Roentgenol 1962;87:171–8.
19. Maxon HR, Thomas SR, Hertzberg VS, et al. Relation between effective radiation dose and outcome of radioiodine therapy for thyroid cancer. N Engl J Med 1983;309:937–41.
20. Jonklaas J, Sarlis NJ, Litofsky D, et al. Outcomes of patients with differentiated thyroid carcinoma following initial therapy. Thyroid 2006;16:1229–42.
21. Bal CS, Kumar A, Chandra P, et al. A prospective clinical trial to assess the efficacy of radioiodine ablation as an alternative to completion thyroidectomy in patients with differentiated thyroid cancer undergoing sub-total thyroidectomy. Acta Oncol 2006; 45:1067–72.
22. Bal C, Padhy AK, Jana S, et al. Prospective randomized clinical trial to evaluate the optimal dose of 131-I for remnant ablation in patients with differentiated thyroid carcinoma. Cancer 1996;77:2574–80.
23. Haugen B, Pacini F, Reiners C, et al. A comparison of recombinant human thyrotropin and thyroid hormone withdrawal for the detection of thyroid remnant or cancer. J Clin Endocrinol Metab 1999;84:3877–85.
24. Schlumberger M, Ricard M, De Pouvourville G, et al. How the availability of recombinant human TSH has changed the management of patients who have thyroid cancer. Nat Clin Pract Endocrinol Metab 2007;3:641–50.
25. Reynolds JC, Robbins J. The changing role of radioiodine in the management of differentiated thyroid cancer. Semin Nucl Med 1997;27:152–64.
26. Hay ID, Grant CS, Taylor WF, et al. Ipsilateral lobectomy versus bilateral lobar resection in papillary thyroid carcinoma: a retrospective analysis of surgical outcome using a novel prognostic scoring system. Surgery 1987;102:1088–95.
27. Hay ID, Grant CS, Bergbstralh EJ, et al. Unilateral total lobectomy: is it sufficient surgical treatment for patients with AMES low-risk papillary thyroid carcinoma? Surgery 1998;124:958–66.
28. Schlumberger M, Berg G, Cohen O, et al. Follow-up of low-risk patients with differentiated thyroid carcinoma: a European perspective. Eur J Endocrinol 2004;150:105–12.
29. Pacini F, Schlumberger M, Dralle H, et al. European consensus for the management of patients with differentiated thyroid carcinoma of the follicular epithelium. Eur J Endocrinol 2006;154:787–803.
30. Baudin E, Schlumberger M. New therapeutic approaches for metastatic thyroid carcinoma. Lancet Oncol 2007;8:148–56.
31. Chaukar DA, Rangarajan V, Nair N, et al. Pediatric thyroid cancer. J Surg Oncol 2005;92:130–3.
32. Chakroborty DK, Bhattacharjee PK, Ray D, et al. Follicular carcinoma of thyroid with synchronous bony and soft tissue metastases. J Indian Med Assoc 2003;101:316–7.
33. Shoup M, Stojadinovic A, Nissan A, et al. Prognostic indicators of outcomes in patients with distant metastases from differentiated thyroid carcinoma. J Am Coll Surg 2003;197:191–7.
34. Mirallié E, Rigaud J, Mathonnet M, et al. Management and prognosis of metastases to the thyroid gland. J Am Coll Surg 2005;200:203–7.
35. Freudenberg LS, Jentzen W, Marlowe RJ, et al. 124-iodine positron emission tomography/computed tomography dosimetry in pediatric patients with differentiated thyroid cancer. Exp Clin Endocrinol Diabetes 2007;115:690–3.
36. Pacini F, Lippi F, Formica N, et al. Therapeutic doses of iodine-131 reveal undiagnosed metastases in thyroid cancer patients with detectable serum thyroglobulin levels. J Nucl Med 1987;28:1888–91.
37. Schlumberger M, Lacroix L, Russo D, et al. Defects in iodide metabolism in thyroid cancer and implications for the follow-up and treatment of patients. Nat Clin Pract Endocrinol Metab 2007;3:260–9.
38. Tuttle RM, Leboeuf R. Investigational therapies for metastatic thyroid carcinoma. J Natl Compr Canc Netw 2007;5:641–6.
39. Ramos CD, Chisin R, Yeung HW, et al. Incidental focal thyroid uptake on FDG positron emission tomographic scans may represent a second primary tumor. Clin Nucl Med 2001;26:193–7.

Surgical Management of Recurrent Thyroid Cancer

Amy Hessel, MD[a,*], Ara A. Chalian, MD[b],
Gary L. Clayman, DMD, MD, FACS[a]

KEYWORDS

- Well differentiated • Recurrent
- Thyroid cancer • Metastasis • Thyroglobulin
- Ultrasound

The prognosis for differentiated thyroid cancer is generally considered excellent with 10-year survival rates greater than 90%.[1] There is widespread agreement that treatment should include surgical thyroidectomy. However, debate continues about the extent of the primary surgery. It is generally accepted for thyroid cancer that clinicians need to assess not only the thyroid gland, but also the regional lymphatics either clinically, radiographically, or intraoperatively. With lymph nodes being palpably present in papillary thyroid carcinoma in up to 15% to 40% of cases and occult in up to 80% of cases,[2] it is important to diagnose those patients who are at risk for regional metastasis. The treatment of the neck in clinically node-positive patients and in high-risk patients is surgery, including the appropriate neck dissection, either central compartment or lateral, depending on the location of the at-risk lymph nodes. If the lateral compartment is involved, ipsilateral central compartment surgery should be considered. Adjuvant therapy with radioactive iodine ablation is considered for high-risk patients, including known residual disease in the thyroid bed, younger patients with distant metastasis (stage II), older patients with large tumors (larger than 1 cm), and is considered for most patients with multifocal disease, nodal metastasis, extrathyroidal or vascular invasion, and aggressive histology.[3]

Despite an aggressive approach to primary differentiated thyroid cancer, a certain percentage of patients develop recurrent disease (5%–20% in papillary and 25%–73% in follicular and Hürthle cell). This can occur either in the thyroid bed or in the lymph nodes, centrally or laterally.[4,5] Because of this propensity for recurrence, it is important to identify which risk factors are involved in recurrent disease, determine how to identify and diagnose recurrent disease, and discuss the treatment options.

RISK FACTORS

Recurrent locoregional disease for differentiated thyroid cancer is relatively common with rates ranging from 5% to 70%. However, despite this, the overall disease 10-year survival is above 90%. This creates a diagnostic and treatment dilemma: How important is it to pursue this disease aggressively when there is already such an excellent long-term outcome? To answer this question, it is necessary to better understand the effect of recurrences on survival and risk of death.

The impact of the development of recurrent disease on long-term survival has been controversial. It is felt that the development of locoregionally recurrent disease increases the risk of death from differentiated thyroid cancer fivefold.[1] Other reports say that while regional recurrence does not adversely affect survival, the development of locorecurrence (primarily thyroid bed) does increase the possibility of tumor-related death in up to 50% of cases.[4] Because of this effect on

---

[a] The Department of Head and Neck Surgery, The University of Texas M. D. Anderson Cancer Center, 1515 Holcombe Boulevard, Box 441, Houston, TX 77030, USA
[b] Department of Otorhinolaryngology: Head and Neck Surgery, University of Pennsylvania Medical Center, 3400 Spruce Street, Philadelphia, PA 19104, USA
* Corresponding author.
E-mail address: ahessel@mdanderson.org (A. Hessel).

overall survival, it becomes important to identify the risk factors that may influence the development of recurrent disease.

Risk Factors for Local Persistent or Recurrent Disease

In patients who develop local disease recurrence, the majority (>50%) of them have stage III (tumors >4 cm) on presentation and are over the age of 45.[4] The type of surgery for the primary disease (hemi-, subtotal, or total thyroidectomy) does not have an impact on the development of thyroid bed recurrences. The development of local recurrence is primarily related to the ability to achieve complete surgical removal of the tumor, regardless of which surgery is used.[1] The presence of central compartment lymph nodes also increases the potential for persistent disease up to 27%.[5]

Risk Factors for Regional Persistent or Recurrent Disease

The development of regional disease after treatment of the primary thyroid cancer can occur in up to 15% of patients.[2] Lymph node metastasis has traditionally not been associated with death from thyroid cancer. However, it is important that the lymph node metastasis be identified during the initial evaluation, and surgical removal at the initial procedure may improve survival. The risk factors for the development of persistent or recurrent disease in the neck include multiple metastatic lymph nodes and extracapsular extension. As reported by Leboulleux and colleagues,[5] when a tumor is less than 4 cm but there are more than 10 metastatic lymph nodes or more than 3 lymph nodes with extracapsular extension, the risk of persistent disease is 20% to 45%. When the metastatic tumor extends above 4 cm, the risk increases to 75%. Recurrent disease follows the same trend, with increased incidence of recurrence when the thyroglobulin is increased and there are multiple lymph nodes and extracapsular extension.

Risk Factors for Decreased Survival

While deaths from differentiated thyroid cancer are rare, some risk factors associated with such deaths can be identified. As discussed in a large matched-control study,[1] the most important risk factor is the completeness of surgical excision of the primary. Incomplete resection of the primary tumor increases both the risk of locoregional recurrence and ultimately the risk of death. In stage III disease, a subtotal resection has a 50% increased risk of death compared with those receiving a total thyroidectomy. However, the extent of lymph node surgery has no impact on overall survival: Those patients receiving extensive modified radical neck dissections tend to have a worse prognosis than those undergoing a lymph node "plucking" procedure, but that prognosis is directly related to increased stage of the disease. The type of adjuvant therapy (radioactive iodine or external beam radiation) does not have any impact on the overall survival of the patients.

As discusses in a large match-control study from Denmark, the overall tumor stage (T4) as well as the diagnosis of distant disease and advanced age are associated with increased risk of death from differentiated thyroid cancer.[6] The overall 5-, 10-, and 15-year survival rates for the patients with T1 through T3 disease is 96%, 93%, and 87%, respectively, while those with T4 disease is 70%, 54%, and 45% respectively. Even more dramatic is the overall survival for the patients with distant disease: 56%, 32%, and 32%.

DIAGNOSIS OF RECURRENCE

After the initial treatment of differentiated thyroid cancer, the patients need long-term follow up and management. Because recurrence of disease is associated with a less favorable prognosis, it becomes important that there be reliable methods for accurate surveillance directed at identifying recurrence in both the primary thyroid bed and the regional nodal basins. The recommended method of follow-up depends on the level of risks for recurrence: low, intermediate, or high. Low-risk patients include those with complete tumor resection and with no local or distant metastasis, no tumor invasion locoregionally, no aggressive histology, no vascular invasion, and no iodine 131 (^{131}I) uptake outside the thyroid bed. The intermediate-risk patients have microscopic extrathyroid invasion, aggressive pathology, and vascular invasion. High-risk patients have macroscopic tumor invasion, incomplete tumor resection, distant metastasis, and ^{131}I uptake outside the thyroid bed (**Box 1**).

Thyroglobulin

Measuring serum thyroglobulin levels is the primary modality of monitoring patients for recurrent or persistent thyroid cancer. Generally, thyroglobulin is a very sensitive and specific method for detecting recurrences. However, differentiated thyroid cancer patients are usually treated with thyroxine replacement, suppressing the thyrotropin below 0.1 mU/L. When thyrotropin is suppressed, the thyroglobulin level is less reliable as a method for detecting small thyroid recurrences. To identify a small recurrence, thyrotropin-stimulation serum thyroglobulin measurements may be required. In addition, if the patient has antithyroglobulin

> **Box 1**
> **Stratification of risk for recurrence of differentiated thyroid cancer**
>
> *Low risk*
> No tumor capsule invasion
> Complete tumor resection
> No vascular invasion
> No aggressive histology
> No ^{131}I uptake outside thyroid bed
> No distant metastasis
>
> *Intermediate risk*
> Microscopic extra thyroid invasion
> Vascular invasion
> Aggressive pathology
>
> *High risk*
> Macroscopic tumor invasion
> Incomplete tumor resection
> ^{131}I uptake outside the thyroid bed
> Distant metastasis

antibodies, the thyroglobulin becomes less sensitive to detect recurrent cancer. While the normal level of thyroglobulin differs for each patient, it is generally accepted that a level above 2 ng/mL is associated with recurrent disease.[3]

Whole-Body Iodine 131 Uptake Scan

A whole-body ^{131}I uptake scan is typically used as a part of the radioactive iodine ablation treatments to determine the accuracy of the ablative procedure. After radioiodine, the whole-body scan is a low sensitivity test (20%)[7] and it is not typically used in low-risk patients, especially if the thyroglobulin is undetectable and the ultrasound is negative. In high-risk patients, a low-dose ^{131}I uptake scan might be useful in evaluations for persistent disease at the 6- to 12-month mark. In the high-risk patient, the low-dose ^{131}I uptake scan, when combined with a stimulated thyroglobulin, offers a sensitivity for identifying recurrent disease approaching 100%.[7]

Cervical Ultrasound

Routine use of high-resolution ultrasound is becoming the main method for postoperative thyroid bed and cervical lymphatic surveillance. As the expertise in this method has improved and as clinicians have become more familiar with the characteristic findings of the postsurgical bed, the sensitivity and specificity of this imaging modality has become very reliable. It is easy to perform and the cost is relatively low. In addition, the ability to perform immediate diagnostic fine needle aspiration on any suspect abnormality makes this a very favorable technique. It is possible to identify recurrences that are as small as 3 to 5 mm.[8] Radiographically, the finding of hypoechoic or cystic mass within the thyroid bed is highly suggestive of recurrence. The identification of further details, such as marginal irregularity, microcalcifications, and taller dimensions, make it possible for ultrasound, in combination with the thyroglobulin test, to deliver a sensitivity of 96% for finding recurrent disease, as compared to 85% when the stimulated thyroglobulin test is used alone.[7] The finding of hypervascular lymph nodes is also very sensitive.

CT

While ultrasound has been traditionally the imaging modality of choice for evaluating the neck for residual or recurrent thyroid cancer, the high-resolution, multislice CT scan can be an important imaging modality for this disease process. It can help identify the location of recurrences and clearly define the anatomic relationships of the paratracheal region, vasculature, and mediastinum. Even more detailed than the standard CT scan, the four-dimensional (4D) CT has been used to offer even more detail to location of the recurrent tumor. The 4D CT scan offers the added dimension of showing changes in perfusion of the contrast over time. The high-resolution images produce excellent documentation of the tumor location and are easily interpreted by surgeons used to reading cross-sectional imaging.[9] The 4D CT scan has been used in parathyroid localization and has proven to be quite useful in delineating the various structures in the thyroid bed and paratracheal region.

The negative aspect of CT is the use of iodinated contrast dye. This iodine load can alter radioactive iodine uptake for 6 weeks.[2] However, in the face of postsurgical thyroid bed recurrences, the benefit of the superior anatomic localization of the 4D CT scan may outweigh the delay in radioiodine administration in regards to successful identification on the tumor in high-risk recurrent thyroid cancer patients. The unenhanced CT scan of the chest can be very sensitive to identify parenchymal disease.

MR Imaging

MR imaging has been an alternative to the iodine-contrasted CT scan for imaging in thyroid cancer. As a cross-sectional imaging study, it has a high sensitivity and accuracy for diagnosing metastatic cervical lymph nodes (95% and 83%, respectively).[10] However, the specificity is only 51% for differentiating between malignant and benign lymph nodes. The use of an MR image for recurrent thyroid cancer can offer excellent information regarding the tumor location and size. However the downsides of MR imaging include the motion artifact that may occur in the paratracheal region, due to respiration; the long length of the study; and the high cost.[2] There is little evidence that imaging with CT or MR image scans in a low-risk primary thyroid cancer increases survival and improves prognosis. However, in the recurrent thyroid cancer patient, the benefit of better tumor localization probably allows for more directed and complete pretreatment planning and surgical procedures.

Fluorine 18 Fluorodeoxyglucose Positron Emission Tomography

In recurrent thyroid cancer patients, the radioactive whole-body scan can be negative in 10% to 15% of patients with detectable serum thyroglobulin levels.[11] This is either because the tumor volume is too small to be seen on iodine scan, or because the thyroid tumor cells are no longer picking up iodine. Because malignancy usually demonstrates increased glucose metabolism, it is likely that the recurrent thyroid cancer lesions that are no longer iodine avid can be visualized on positron emission tomography (PET–CT) scan. Several studies have demonstrated sensitivities of PET–CT scanning for identifying recurrent or metastatic thyroid cancer in the range of 66% to 79%.[1,11,12] The combined PET–CT scan is most useful in the situation of low thyroglobulin (<10 ng/mL) and poor or no iodine concentration on whole-body imaging. When the PET–CT scan is positive, it can be very helpful in localizing the area of recurrent tumor and assist in surgical planning.

However, PET–CT scan is not useful as a screening tool because the false-negative rates are relatively high (15%–30%).[11–13] Instead, the PET–CT scan should be used as an adjunct to the conventional imaging (ultrasound and whole-body scan) and fine needle aspiration. In addition, the PET–CT scan has been accurate in diagnosing subtle lung metastasis (>6 mm) and should be considered when there is elevated thyroglobulin and no iodine uptake on whole body imaging. See **Table 1** for summary.

TREATMENT OF RECURRENT WELL-DIFFERENTIATED THYROID CANCER

The treatment algorithm of recurrent or metastatic well-differentiated thyroid cancer should be

Table 1
A suggested algorithm for the use of imaging in detecting recurrent thyroid cancer

	Ultrasound	Whole-Body Scan	CT	MR Imaging	PET–CT
Preoperation	++++ ☒Operator dependent	—	+ ☑Localization ☒Iodine	++ ☑No iodine	—
Postoperation before radioiodine	++	++++ ☑Pre-tx evaluation	—	—	—
Follow-up (thyroglobulin low)	++++	—	—	—	—
Follow-up (thyroglobulin elevated)	++++	+++	++ ☑Localization	++ ☑Localization ☒Motion artifact	+ ☒High false negative
Locoregional recurrence	++++	+	++++ ☑Localization	++ ☑Localization ☒Motion artifact	++ ☑Localization
Distant metastasis	—	+++ ☑If iodine sensitive	—	—	+++ ☑Small pulmonary metastasis

Symbols: +, sometimes useful; ++, usually useful; +++, very useful; ++++, essential; —, not useful; ☒, drawback; ☑, advantage.

prioritized to surgical excision of locoregional disease (for those patients who can be cured), ^{131}I therapy, external beam radiation, watchful waiting for those with stable disease, and experimental chemotherapy.[3] The development of recurrence and the extent of disease both have an impact on tumor-related mortality with rates of 10% for local recurrence, 36% for regional recurrence, 50% for locoregional recurrence, and 100% for distant metastasis.[4]

Surgical Management of Thyroid Remnant, Thyroid Bed, and Central Compartment

Surgery is the preferred treatment modality of resectable recurrent thyroid carcinoma. The majority of locally recurrent tumors occur in the thyroid bed or in the thyroid remnant. In either case, surgical resection is called for. However, there is a distinct difference in resectability depending on the location of the recurrence: 90% in a thyroid remnant versus 45% in the thyroid bed.[4] This is important because disease-free survival is linked to the ability to completely resect the recurrent disease with thyroid bed recurrence disease-specific survival of 45% while thyroid remnant recurrence disease-specific survival is 85%.

Surgery for the thyroid bed should be performed after localization of the tumor has been obtained on imaging (ultrasound, CT, PET–CT). The surgical goal is complete resection of the residual or recurrent thyroid tissue with preservation of the recurrent laryngeal nerve and parathyroids when possible. It is important to document the preoperative mobility of the vocal folds either with direct mirror examination of the larynx or with fiber-optic laryngoscopy.

The surgical approach to the thyroid bed should include identification and protection of the recurrent laryngeal nerves. In the previously operated thyroid bed, the nerve is often contained within fibrotic scar and can be somewhat difficult to identify. It has been suggested that the use of intraoperative recurrent laryngeal nerve monitoring via the endotracheal tube can be useful in identification.[14] However, it is important that the nerve monitor not take the place of good surgical technique and knowledge of the anatomy. Before the surgical procedure, it is again important to document vocal fold mobility with fiber-optic laryngoscopy to assist with preoperative counseling, surgical planning, and anticipation of potentially invasive disease.

The surgical approach to the thyroid bed and central compartment should be done through the prior incision site. All attempts should be made to maintain the current anatomy. However, due to heavy scarring and fibrosis, it may be necessary to remove the overlying strap muscles to gain good visualization of the thyroid bed. Other strategies to decrease the risk of injury to the recurrent laryngeal nerve include identifying the nerve low in the tracheoesophageal groove well below the thyroid bed and performing an inferior-to-superior dissection for the central compartment dissection.[15] The approach of following the carotid artery inferiorly also allows dissection in potential unscarred planes to assist in recurrent laryngeal nerve identification.

The central compartment dissection should contain all of the remaining lymphatic tissue from the carotid artery laterally to the trachea medially. Superiorly, the dissection should extend from the just above the cricoid to the level of the clavicle inferiorly. Most dissections stop at or in the superior thymus, especially as this often allows for the inferior parathyroid to be preserved. These boundaries, however, are also determined by the location of the known recurrent disease. Each reoperation should be tailored to safely remove all of the respectable disease within the neck. "Berry picking" of the affected lymph nodes should be avoided. Instead the focus should be on identifying the appropriate anatomy and removing the at-risk and involved levels of lymph nodes. Elective dissection of the neck, central compartment, or thyroid bed where there is no documented disease should be avoided to decrease the risks. In the face of heavy scar formation, it may be difficult to locate the recurrent disease, especially when the tumor is less than 20 mm. The use of intraoperative ultrasound has been found to be very helpful in localizing the disease.[16,17]

The risk of reoperation in the thyroid bed and central compartment carries increased risks to both the recurrent laryngeal nerve and to the remaining parathyroid glands when compared with primary surgery in this area. The risk of recurrent laryngeal nerve injury resulting in permanent vocal cord paralysis ranges from 1% to 12%, which is higher than the risk in primary thyroid surgery (1%–5%).[15] If the tumor adheres to the nerve but can be dissected away, the nerve should preserved. Resection of the nerve may be required if the tumor encompasses the nerve. The parathyroid glands in revision central compartment surgery are at high risk for devascularization and inadvertent removal because the anatomic location of the glands is no longer predictable. The incidence of permanent hypoparathyroidism after reoperation ranges from 1% to 4%.[15] All attempts to identify the parathyroid glands pathologically should be done and, if there is concern about the viability, they should be reimplanted either in the local muscles of the head and neck (sternocleidomastoid is most common) or the arm if the neck is compromised by prior radiation therapy or multiple recurrent lateral neck disease.

Surgical Management of Laryngotracheal Invasion

In regards to the thyroid bed, it is not uncommon for the recurrent disease to adhere to the tracheal or esophageal wall or to minimally invading the tracheal or esophageal wall. Laryngeal or tracheal invasion can be found in around 4% to 16% of patients and has been found to be an independent predictor of poor prognosis.[18,19] Symptoms that may indicate invasion include hemoptysis, hoarseness, and dyspnea. However, minor involvement may be completely asymptomatic. Preoperative anatomic imaging (CT scan) can be very helpful in predicting airway involvement and should be considered for the symptomatic patient. If there is gross invasion that may require a tracheal resection, a bronchoscopy before surgery may be helpful in perioperative planning. The length of tracheal resection necessary must be determined beforehand to make sure a primary anastomosis is possible. If a primary anastomosis is not possible, then a mediastinal tracheostomy will be required.

Complete resection has been directly tied to improved prognosis and successful palliation, even in the face of pulmonary metastasis. Patients who underwent radical resection with complete tumor removal were able to achieve a 5-year survival rate of abut 77% and a 10-year survival rate of about 60%,[20] while those with residual disease after resection had 5-year survivals of just over 20%.[19] Therefore, all attempts should be made to remove the invaded structure. It has been suggested that the extent of radical resection makes no difference in survival as long as complete tumor resection is achieved. Thus, a tumor with minimal tracheal invasion treated with a shave resection will achieve the same result in regards to tumor control as a tumor with gross invasion of the airway undergoing a complete tracheal resection, as long as the entire tumor was removed.[18,19]

The surgeon should seek out surgical resection options that offer the lowest perioperative morbidity and the highest long-term quality of life. This means weighing the benefits and drawbacks of various surgical procedures for laryngotracheal involvement. Among such procedures are shave resection of the tracheal or cricoid, complete tracheal resection, resection of esophageal musculature, and total laryngectomy or laryngopharyngectomy. With each surgical procedure, the appropriate reconstruction must be considered.

For a small defect created from a shave resection of cricoid or trachea, a watertight closure can be reconstructed with a patch of soft tissue, such as strap muscle, sternocleidomastoid muscle, or pectoralis muscle rotational flap. If a full segment of trachea (up to about 5 cm) must be removed, then a primary end-to-end anastomosis is appropriate. In very long defects in the trachea, reconstruction is much more complex. In the past, these long defects have resulted in a laryngectomy with tracheal resection and a mediastinal stoma. Recently, case reports have appeared describing the use of vascularized free flaps, such as the radial forearm free-tissue transfer with prosthesis stenting.[21] For large tracheal defects, a challenge for surgeons is to create rigid support for airway maintenance and a soft tissue closure that will allow for re-epithelialization and secretion clearance.

As with any laryngotracheal surgery, airway management must be of primary concern. The use of tracheostomy should be discussed in all cases requiring laryngotracheal resection. The indications for intraoperative tracheostomy should include the loss of the supporting structures of the airway, the possibility of prolonged postoperative edema, and significant dissection (or sacrifice) of the recurrent laryngeal nerves causing potential for temporary or permanent vocal fold paralysis.

In those patients with gross laryngeal and upper tracheal involvement, specifically around the cricothyroid membrane and cricoid cartilage, the risk for permanent airway compromise due to bilateral vocal cord fixation or an incompetent larynx resulting in aspiration and feeding tube dependence, total laryngectomy (or laryngopharyngectomy) should be considered. In this setting, voice rehabilitation with primary or secondary tracheoesophageal puncture should be offered. In the setting of a laryngopharyngectomy, soft tissue free-flap reconstruction of the pharynx should be planned.

Surgical resection and reconstruction of the laryngotracheal structure for recurrent thyroid carcinoma carries a relatively high risk of complications (up to 39%), including unilateral or bilateral vocal cord paralysis (8%), transient hypoparathyroidism (10%–50%), permanent hypoparathyroidism (3%–9%), temporary tracheostomy (18%), permanent tracheostomy (4%), anastomotic leak (4%–6%), and dysphagia/aspiration (3%–7%).[18–20] Clearly the development of these complications is highly dependent on the presenting disease status as well as the location and invasiveness of the recurrent thyroid disease. These procedures carry a perioperative death risk ranging between 1% and 4%.[15,18,19]

Surgical Management of the Lateral Neck

Identification of recurrent disease in the lateral neck is often found on ultrasound imaging of the neck in follow-up. Once identified, fine needle aspiration can be used to diagnose the presence of regional metastasis. Due to the high incidence of multiple lymph node involvement, it is important to address surgically the entire nodal basin and avoid "berry picking." In the face of lateral neck metastasis, an anatomic radiographic imaging study is often useful to identify the critical structures and to plan the neck dissection.

The removal of the lymph nodes should be done with a selective neck dissection, preserving the nononcologic structures whenever possible. There is no role for elective modified radical or radical neck dissection. Instead, the jugular vein, spinal accessory nerve, and sternocleidomastoid muscle should be left intact unless directly invaded by an aggressive nodal metastasis. The lymph nodes removed should include the highest involved nodal basin and then the drainage basin below. For example, nodal metastases within level II can be dissected with a selective neck dissection including levels II, III, and IV. A posterior lymph node in lower level V can be dissected with levels IV, V, and the ipsilateral VI.

In recurrent thyroid cancer, elective removal of the contralateral lymph nodes is not indicated. It is important that the entire neck be evaluated before surgery to know exactly which nodal basins are suspicious for recurrent disease. The use of intraoperative ultrasound can be helpful in the case of indeterminate nodules seen on preoperative imaging, or in patients who have difficult anatomy from prior treatment (surgery and radiotherapy).[16] The goal of lateral neck dissection is complete surgical removal of the malignant nodes with low morbidity. The risk of complications associated with neck dissection is rare. The nature of the potential complications depends on the levels dissected. Potential complications include injury to the greater auricular nerve (ear numbness), injury to the spinal accessory nerve (shoulder dysfunction), injury to the marginal mandibular nerve (lower lip weakness), injury to the hypoglossal nerve (tongue weakness), injury to the vagus nerve (hoarseness), injury to the phrenic nerve (diaphragm elevation), and injury to the brachial plexus (arm weakness and numbness).[2]

ROLE OF EXTERNAL BEAM RADIATION IN RECURRENT THYROID CANCER

The use of radiation for well-differentiated thyroid cancer has been controversial in all fields that treat thyroid cancer, especially in those patients who are being treated for the primary thyroid disease. However, the use of radiation has been more common in the area of recurrent thyroid cancer. For recurrences in the lateral neck, surgery with radioablative iodine therapy has been the standard of care. However, external beam radiation is often considered after recurrence in the neck when surgical resection reveals soft tissue involvement or extracapsular extension on pathology. In regards to recurrent disease in the thyroid bed, external beam radiation should be considered if there is gross extension outside of the residual thyroid gland.[22]

External beam radiation to this area carries side effects and morbidity, and the overall effect on locoregional recurrence and survival has not been clearly shown to be positive. Thus, this treatment modality is often saved for the recurrent disease in which further surgical management (with or without radioactive iodine) will compromise function, diminish quality of life, or be likely ineffective.[3,22]

SUMMARY

While well-differentiated thyroid cancer is generally thought to be a treatable cancer with excellent outcomes in regards to locoregional control and survival, some patients suffer from recurrent disease and possible decreased overall prognosis. Identifying those patients who are high risk for recurrent disease is often difficult. Risk factors for recurrent disease include primary disease greater than 4 cm, incomplete resection, multiple positive lymph nodes in the central compartment, and lateral neck disease with multiple positive lymph nodes in multiple levels or pathologic extracapsular extension. These factors can help stratify the thyroid cancer population into low-, medium-, and high-risk patients.

The low-risk patients (those with completely resected tumor without adverse pathology or invasion, no thyroid uptake outside the thyroid bed, and no distant metastasis) can generally be followed with thyroglobulin levels and routine ultrasounds to the head and neck. The high-risk patients (those with macroscopic tumor invasion, incomplete tumor resection, distant metastasis, and ^{131}I uptake outside the thyroid bed) are best monitored with stimulated thyroglobulin, ultrasound of the head and neck, and low-dose ^{131}I uptake scans at the 6- to 12-month mark. Four-dimensional CT scans and MR image scans are used for anatomic localization of suspected thyroid cancer recurrences.

The role of 18F-fluoro-deoxy-glucose PET, in the diagnosis and identification of recurrent thyroid cancer is still evolving. At this point, the PET–CT scan is most useful in the situation of low thyroglobulin (<10 ng/mL) and poor or no iodine concentration on whole-body imaging in the high-risk patient. While not used as a screening tool, it can be used as an adjunct to the conventional imaging (ultrasound and whole-body scan) and fine needle aspiration or in the setting elevated thyroglobulin and no iodine uptake on whole-body imaging.

The treatment of locoregional recurrent thyroid cancer remains surgical resection whenever possible. All attempts at complete tumor removal should be made, keeping in mind the increased risk for complications, such as recurrent laryngeal nerve injury and hypoparathryoidism. Surgical resection should include the location in which there is identified tumor (thyroid bed, central compartment, or lateral neck) but avoiding elective dissection of the noninvolved lymph node compartments. With complete tumor excision remaining the goal of surgery, the involved tissues should be removed, including the appropriate neck dissection; the central compartment cleaned out; and, if necessary, the laryngotracheal complex resected. Reconstruction should be directed to maintaining a patent and safe airway as well as preserving function. Reoperation after prior treatment for thyroid cancer can be risky, and the appropriate counseling must be done with the patient preoperatively.

Adjuvant therapy after surgery for recurrent thyroid cancer is often necessary. Radioactive iodine should be given whenever possible. However, if it is unlikely that surgery and radioiodine will be successful in maintaining recurrence-free status, external beam radiation should be considered.

It is well understood that the development of recurrent thyroid cancer after effective therapy results in a decrease in further locoregional control as well as overall survival. So, the goal of therapy should focus on complete a tumor resection as well as the maintenance of function.

REFERENCES

1. Lundgren CI, Hall P, Dickman PW, et al. Influence of surgical and postoperative treatment on survival in differentiated thyroid cancer. Br J Surg 2007;94:571–7.
2. Watkinson J, Franklyn JA, Olliff JFC. Detection and surgical treatment of cervical lymph nodes in differentiated thyroid cancer. Thyroid 2006;16(2):187–94.
3. Cooper DS, Doherty GM, Haugen BR, et al. Management guidelines for patients with thyroid nodules and differentiated thyroid cancer. Thyroid 2006;16(2):109–42.
4. Stojadinovic A, Shoup M, Nissan A, et al. Recurrent differentiated thyroid carcinoma: biological implications of age, method of detection and site and extent of recurrence. Ann Surg Oncol 2002;9(8):789–98.
5. Leboulleux S, Rubino C, Baudin E, et al. Prognostic factors for persistent or recurrent disease of papillary thyroid carcinoma with neck lymph node metastases and/or extension beyond the thyroid capsule at initial diagnosis. J Clin Endocrinol Metab 2005;90(10):5723–9.
6. Eustatia-Rutten CFA, Corssmit EPM, Biermasz NR, et al. Survival and death causes in differentiated thyroid carcinoma. J Clin Endocrinol Metab 2006;91(1):313–9.
7. Pacini F, Molinaro E, Castagna G, et al. Recombinant human thyrotropin–stimulated serum thyroglobulin combined with neck ultrasonography has the highest sensitivity in monitoring differentiated thyroid carcinoma. J Clin Endocrinol Metab 2003;88:3668–78.
8. Lee JH, Lee HK, Lee DH, et al. Ultrasonoraphic findings of a newly detected nodule on the thyroid bed in postoperative patients for thyroid carcinoma: correlation with the results of ultrasonography-guided fine needle aspiration biopsy. Clin Imaging 2007;31:109–31.
9. Rogers SE, Hunter GJ, Hamberg LM, et al. Improved preoperative planning for directed parathyroidectomy with 4-dimensional computed tomography. Surgery 2006;140:932–41.
10. Gross ND, Weissman JL, Talbot M, et al. MRI detection of cervical metastasis from differentiated thyroid carcinoma. Laryngoscope 2001;111:1905–9.
11. Shamas M, Begirmenci B, Mountz JM, et al. ^{18}F-FDG PET/CT in patients with suspected recurrent or metastatic well-differentiated thyroid cancer. J Nucl Med 2007;48(2):221–6.
12. Palemdo H, Bucerius J, Joe A, et al. Integrated PET/CT in differentiated thyroid cancer: diagnostic accurate and impact on patient management. J Nucl Med 2006;47(4):616–24.
13. Nahas S, Golenlberg D, Fakhry C, et al. The role of positron emission tomography/computed tomography in the management of recurrent papillary thyroid carcinoma. Laryngoscope 2005;115:237–43.
14. Farrag TY, Agrwal N, Sheth S, et al. Algorithm of safe and effective reoperative thyroid bed surgery for recurrent/persistent thyroid carcinoma. Head Neck 2007, in press.
15. Kim MK, Mandel SH, Baloch Z, et al. Morbidity following central compartment preoperation for recurrent or persistent thyroid cancer. Arch Otolaryngol Head Neck Surg 2004;130:1214–6.
16. Karwowski JK, Jeffery RB, McDougall IR, et al. Intraoperative ultrasonography improves identification of recurrent thyroid cancer. Surgery 2002;132:924–9.
17. Ishigaki A, Shimamoto K, Satake H, et al. Multi-slice CT of thyroid nodules: comparison with ultrasonography. Radiat Med 2004;22(5):346–53.

18. Gaissert HA, Honings J, Grillo HC, et al. Segmental laryngotracheal and tracheal resection for invasive thyroid carcinoma. Ann Thorac Surg 2007;83:1952–9.
19. Kowalski LP, Filho JG. Results of the treatment of locally invasive thyroid carcinoma. Head Neck 2002;24(4):340–4.
20. Nakao K, Kurosumi K, Fukushima S, et al. Merits and demerits of operative procedure to the trachea in patients with differentiated thyroid cancer. World J Surg 2001;25:723–7.
21. Yu P, Clayman G, Walsh G. Human tracheal reconstruction with a composite radial forearm free flap and prosthesis. Ann Thorac Surg 2006;81:714–6.
22. Lee N, Tuttle M. The role of external beam radiotherapy in the treatment of papillary thyroid cancer. Endocr Relat Cancer 2006;13:971–7.

Extrathyroidal Manifestations of Thyroid Disease: Thyroid Ophthalmopathy

Hemant Parmar, MD*, Mohannad Ibrahim, MD

KEYWORDS

- Thyroid ophthalmopathy • Graves disease • Imaging

Graves disease or thyroid ophthalmopathy (TO) is an autoimmune disease affecting the thyroid gland, orbital soft tissues, and subcutaneous tissues of the extremities. It is the most common type of hyperthyroidism, which is a state of excess circulating thyroid hormones attributable to overstimulation and oversecretion of the thyroid gland. It differs from thyrotoxicosis, which is a state of excess circulating thyroid hormones irrespective of the cause. It was in 1835 that Robert Graves described four cases of ophthalmopathy associated with thyroid disease.[1] Although in recent years the disease has been called by Graves's name, the first original description of the disease was made by Caleb Perry around 1825. Karl von Basedow later described the association of exophthalmos and thyrotoxicosis. This disorder thus is sometimes also referred as Parry disease or von Basedow disease.[1,2] Our understanding of TO has greatly increased in the last 2 decades, but several issues regarding nomenclature, pathophysiology, and treatment are yet to be completely elucidated. Fundamentally, there is still disagreement over the correct name and it is referred to by many names, such as thyroid-associated ophthalmopathy, autoimmune thyroid disease, endocrine exophthalmos, malignant exophthalmos, dysthyroid ophthalmopathy, and thyroid eye disease. Graves disease is the most commonly used name in United States.[3]

TO has an approximate incidence of 0.5% in United States.[4] It is one of the common orbital disorders and is the underlying cause in 15% to 28% of unilateral exophthalmos and almost 80% of bilateral exophthalmos.[5–7] Approximately 70% to 80% of patients who have TO develop hyperthyroidism within an 18-month period.[8] A small percentage of patients have hypothyroidism or Hashimoto thyroiditis together with eye signs.[9]

PATHOLOGY AND PATHOPHYSIOLOGY

On histopathology the most prominent finding in TO is swelling of the extraocular muscles (EOMs), which can become grossly enlarged.[10] In postmortem work, Rundle and colleagues[11] analyzed the EOM in a man who had severe TO who died of myocardial infarction. The swollen EOM felt like rubber and had a diameter of greater than 1 cm. On microscopy the muscles showed fibrosis, edema, and lymphocytic infiltration. The swelling of the muscles was not because of an increase in the number of muscle fibers, but because of an increase in the volume of individual fibers plus an increase in connective tissue. Separately, using three-dimensional CT volume studies, van der Gaag and colleagues[12] found swelling of EOMs alone in 20% of their patients who had TO. In 48% both EOMs and the adipose tissues were swollen, whereas in 28% the EOM volume was normal but the adipose tissue compartment had increased in volume; in 4% an increase in orbital tissue was apparent. It therefore appears that fat,

Division of Neuroradiology, Department of Radiology, University of Michigan Health System, University of Michigan, 1500 East Medical Center Drive, Ann Arbor, MI 48109-0302, USA
* Corresponding author.
E-mail address: hparmar@umich.edu (H. Parmar).

muscles, and the lacrimal gland can increase considerably in volume in patients who have TO.

In the earlier descriptions it was noticed that the swelling of the EOMs and adipose tissue was attributable to an increase in what was called the "ground substance." Now we know that this substance consists of collagen and glycosaminoglycans (GAGs), which can be found throughout the muscle fibers in the endomysial space.[13] The most prominently present GAGs are hyaluronic acid and chondroitin sulfate. GAGs are hydrophilic and thus attract water and cause edema of the EOMs and retro-ocular tissues. Despite this accumulation of GAGs and collagen there is no evidence of damage to the muscle fibers themselves.[14] In addition many researchers have found deposition of fibroblasts within the endomysial space and in the connective/adipose tissues, which are considered to be responsible for the overproduction of GAG. Apart from these fibroblasts, there is also a mononuclear cell infiltration, consisting of lymphocytes, macrophages, and plasma cells. The chronic stage of TO results in interstitial fibrosis with resultant muscle atrophy and fatty degeneration.[15] Electron microscopy and electromyography have not detected a primary pathologic process in the muscle cells, confirming that the degeneration and atrophy are secondary to interstitial inflammation and fibrosis.[16]

The fundamental cause of TO is the production of autoantibodies that bind to and stimulate the thyroid-stimulating hormone receptor (TSHR). The close clinical association between autoimmune hyperthyroidism, ophthalmopathy, and pretibial dermopathy suggests that the antigen responsible for these diverse conditions is common to the thyroid gland, orbital tissues, and pretibial skin.[17,18] It is postulated that the immune complexes reach the orbit by way of the superior cervical lymph channels that drain the thyroid gland and the orbit.[19] Although the exact cause for TO remains unknown, the disease is believed to result from a complex interplay of genetic and environmental factors.[20] Genes, such as those for human leukocyte antigen, may determine a patient's susceptibility to the disease and its severity, but environmental factors, often unknown, determine its course. Once established the inflammatory process within the orbital tissues seems to take on a momentum of its own. Based on this current state of knowledge it is proposed[20] that in patients who have TO the circulating T cells, directed against certain antigens on thyroid follicular cells, recognize epitopes of antigens following processing and presentation by dendritic cells and non-professional antigen-presenting cells, such as orbital fibroblasts. Orbital preadipocytes and fibroblasts are stimulated by unknown circulating or locally produced factors to differentiate into mature adipocytes that express increased levels of TSHR. T cell recruitment into orbital tissues is facilitated by various cytokines and chemokines, which help to attract T cells by stimulating the expression of certain adhesion molecules (eg, ICAM-1, VAM-1, CD44). T cells and macrophages along with local fibroblasts and adipocytes are known to synthesize and release several cytokines (most likely Th-1 type spectrum) into the surrounding tissues. Cytokines, oxygen free radicals, and fibrogenic growth factors, released from infiltrating inflammatory and residential cells, act on orbital preadipocytes to stimulate adipogenesis, fibroblast proliferation, GAG synthesis, and expression of immunomodulatory molecules. Smoking, a well-known aggravating factor for TO, may enhance tissue hypoxia and exert immunomodulatory effects. The long-held hypothesis of thyroid cross-reactive or shared antigen with the orbital tissues has recently gained significant support from animal models and by in vitro and ex vivo studies.[20]

CLINICAL FEATURES

Depending on the intake of iodine, TO forms 50% to 60% of hyperthyroidism in Europe and is the most common autoimmune disease in United States.[21] Its incidence is 0.5:1000 women per year.[4] The signs and symptoms of TO are varied and involve different systems. Symptoms of hyperthyroidism often result in changes in energy level, weight, sleep, bowel movements, heart rate, heart rhythm, skin, and hair. Family history is helpful because TO is believed to have more than 30% identifiable heredity along with other autoimmune disorders.[9] Although it can occur over a wide age range of 15 to 86 years, it typically peaks in the fourth and fifth decades of life. Females are affected much more than males, in the ratio of 4 to 1. Social history is sometimes helpful because it is known to be aggravated by smoking, stress, dietary factors, and other extraneous factors.[9]

The main clinical features of TO are summarized in Werner Classification, known as NOSPECS[19,22] (**Table 1**).

Class I: Only Signs, No Symptoms

This class refers to upper eyelid retraction. This retraction causes stare and lid lag on downward gaze (von Graefe sign) and can be caused by swelling of the superior levator muscle. Early in the disease this lid retraction is sympathomimetic

Table 1
Classification of eye changes of thyroid ophthalmopathy: the NO SPECS classification

Class	Grade	Suggestions for Grading
0		No physical signs or symptoms
1		Only signs
2		Soft tissue involvement
	0	Absent
	a	Minimal
	b	Moderate
	c	Marked
3		Proptosis 3 mm or more above upper normal limit
	0	Absent
	a	23–24 mm
	b	25–27 mm
	c	>28 mm
4		EOM involvement: graded according to diplopia
	0	Absent
	a	Intermittent (when fatigued)
	b	Inconstant (at extremes of gaze)
	c	Constant (in primary gaze)
5		Corneal involvement
	0	Absent
	a	Stippling of cornea
	b	Ulceration
	c	Clouding, necrosis, perforation
6		Vision loss attributable to optic nerve involvement
	0	Absent
	a	Disc pallor, visual field defect, vision 0.63–0.5
	b	Same, but vision is 0.4–0.1
	c	Same, but vision <0.1–blindness

Data from Werner SC. Modification of the classification of the eye changes of Graves' disease: recommendations of the ad hoc committee of the American Thyroid Association. J Clin Endocrinol Metab 1977;44:203–4.

but in later stages it is attributable to fibrosis of the lid tissue.[23,24]

Class II: Soft Tissue Involvement

This class entails chemosis (edema of the conjunctiva), conjunctival injection, and redness and swollen upper and lower eyelids. These findings are partly explained by impaired venous drainage because of an increase in retrobulbar tissue.[25] Another explanation for the swelling of the eyelids is herniation of retrobulbar tissue through the naturally occurring herniations in the orbital septum.[26,27]

Class III: Proptosis

Because of confining bony walls, the swollen retrobulbar tissue has no other outlet than pushing the globe forward. In postmortem studies Rundle and Pochin demonstrated that the normal orbital volume of eye muscles is 3.5 mL and the orbital cavity is 26 mL.[28] They then showed that an increase in muscle volume of 4 mL causes a proptosis of 6 mm. Small change in tissue volume can thus cause considerable proptosis.

Class IV: Extraocular Muscle Involvement

With increasing swelling, there is impairment in the normal motility of the EOMs. Motility disturbances are also seen with thyroid ophthalmopathy. It is initially characterized by limitation of lid elevation followed by limitation in horizontal movement. These limitations are usually associated with diplopia in the corresponding visual fields. Although all muscles at some stage may be involved in the disease process, the order of involvement is inferior rectus muscles followed by medial, superior, and lateral recti.

Class V: Corneal Involvement

Exophthalmos, lid retraction, and less frequent blinking all contribute to exposure of the cornea, which can lead to keratitis. Early signs are photophobia, a gritty sensation, blurred vision, and intolerance to contact lenses. The presence of corneal irritation is not by itself a sign of severe ophthalmopathy, because it can be relieved by liberal application of eye drops and ointments.

Class VI: Vision Loss

Vision loss because of optic nerve damage can be combined with visual field defects and impaired color vision.[29] There is no evidence of direct inflammation of the optic nerve itself and optic neuropathy is probably attributable to swelling and compression from EOMs or venous stasis close to the apex of the orbit, known as apical crowding. Another explanation is an increase in retrobulbar pressure.

Dolman and colleagues[30] advocated VISA classification for patients who have thyroid ophthalmopathy. The VISA acronym stands for vision, inflammation, strabismus, and appearance/exposure, and deals with four common dysfunctions of TO.

DIAGNOSIS AND ROLE OF IMAGING

The diagnosis of TO is based primarily on the patient's presenting symptoms and findings on clinical examination. Laboratory testing and imaging studies are valuable in confirming the diagnosis. Exophthalmos, lid retraction, lid lag, prominence of episcleral vessels, and lid edema are important clinical findings. In some patients the disease manifests as gradual onset of vertical gaze diplopia.[31] On examination there is exophthalmos. It is usually bilateral and symmetric; however, asymmetric and unilateral forms of exophthalmos are also seen.[32] Ultrasound of the orbit reveals irregularity with medium to high reflectivity on A-scan. On B-scan there is enlargement of the EOM bellies with sparing of the tendons. The superior ophthalmic vein can be enlarged and Doppler examination shows increased arterial flow.[3]

IMAGING

The diagnosis of thyroid ophthalmopathy is mainly clinical. Imaging is preferred for evaluation of cases in which the diagnosis is uncertain.[33] At our institute CT is usually the preferred modality of imaging for disease; MR imaging does not offer significant advantages over CT, except for evaluation of the optic nerve. CT is used to assess EOM enlargement, fatty expansion, and optic nerve compression, especially before surgery and as a follow-up after treatment. CT is usually performed using 2.5-mm thick sections in both axial and coronal planes and study is often obtained with intravenous contrast media. Typically, enlargement of the EOM involves the belly of the muscle and spares the anterior tendinous insertions; rarely there could be thickening of the tendinous portions.[34] In the initial stages this enlargement can be subtle (**Fig. 1**). The enlarged EOM shows low density as a result of focal accumulation of lymphocytes and mucopolysaccharide accumulation (**Fig. 2**).[34] On MR imaging the involved muscle shows low signal on T1-weighted image (WI) (**Fig. 3**A) and intermediate to high signal on T2 WI (**Fig. 3**B). There is marked enhancement of the EOMs following gadolinium-based contrast agent (**Fig. 3**C) because of increased vascularity of the EOMs allowing for diffusion of contrast material into the muscular tissue. Although patients can show unilateral involvement clinically, bilateral CT and MR imaging abnormalities are seen in approximately 90% of cases.[34] Bilateral involvement may be either asymmetric (**Fig. 4**A) or symmetric (**Fig. 4**B). Sometimes with progress of disease and clinical symptoms there

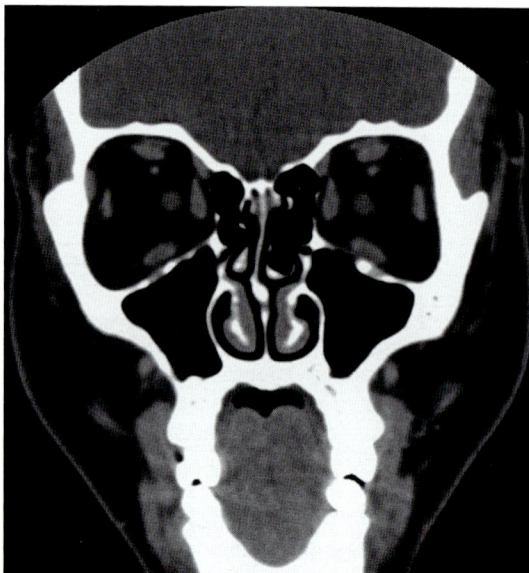

Fig. 1. Thyroid ophthalmopathy with early muscle involvement. Coronal CT section through the mid-orbit reveal subtle enlargement of bilateral medial and inferior rectus muscles. There is also mild hazy appearance of the retro-ocular fat.

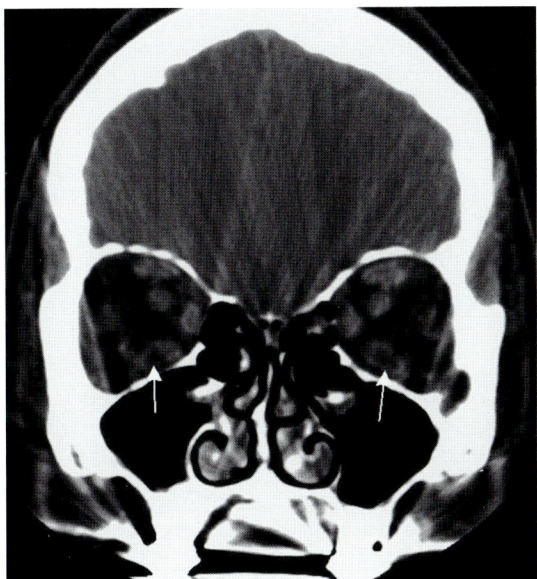

Fig. 2. Thyroid ophthalmopathy with moderate enlargement of muscles. Coronal CT sections of the mid-orbit show bilateral symmetric involvement of the inferior, medial, and superior rectus muscles. Note hypodensities within bilateral inferior rectus muscles suggestive of deposition of lymphocytes and mucopolysaccharides (*arrows*).

is progression of the muscle involvement over time (**Fig. 5**A, B). In order of frequency, the inferior rectus is the most common muscle involved followed by medial rectus muscle and superior muscle complex (composed of superior rectus and levator palpebral muscles); sometimes the superior oblique muscle is involved (see **Fig. 3**). The lateral rectus muscle enlargement is less pronounced and in most cases it appears normal. The degree of enlargement varies from mild to severe; in severe cases a significant portion of the orbital space is obliterated by enlarged muscles. Significant muscle enlargement can exert extrinsic pressure on the optic nerve at the orbital apex and can lead to visual field defects and vision loss (**Fig. 6**). It has been shown that increased volume of the EOMs correlates with the severity of optic neuropathy.[35,36] Furthermore, improvement of optic neuropathy seems to correlate with a decrease in EOM swelling. Significant enlargement of the muscle can lead to remodeling of the adjacent bones, especially the thin lamina papyracea.[9] The second common finding in TO is expansion of the retro-ocular fat resulting in proptosis (**Fig. 7**). Fatty expansion can lead to considerable stretching and strengthening of the optic nerves. Other imaging findings in TO include increased density or stranding within the retro-ocular fat, which has been shown to be caused by increased lymphocytic proliferation and vascular congestion (**Fig. 8**A, B). In some cases there can be enlargement of the lacrimal glands because of increased lymphocytic infiltration, edema (chemosis) of the eyelids, and anterior displacement of the orbital septum.

In the late or chronic phase of the disease there is a decrease in muscle swelling and the muscles appear more atrophic (**Fig. 9**A). There are restricted eye movements secondary to fibrosis of the EOMs and subsequent loss of elasticity.[31] At this stage CT and MR imaging show fatty replacement of the EOMs (**Fig. 9**B). Although the muscles are attenuated, the retro-ocular fat volume remains increased.

DIFFERENTIAL DIAGNOSIS

Several other entities that can result in enlargement of the EOMs include orbital pseudotumor,

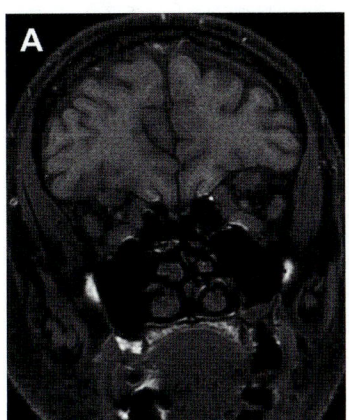 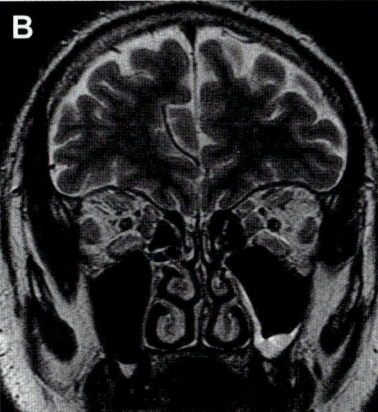 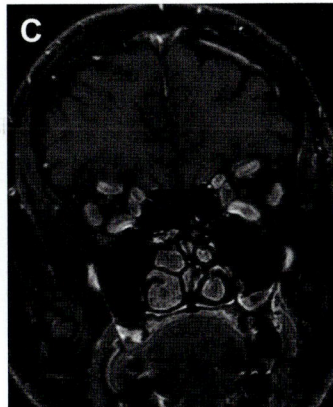

Fig. 3. Thyroid ophthalmopathy with MR imaging of bilateral muscle enlargement. Coronal T1 WI (*A*), T2 WI (*B*), and post–contrast-enhanced (*C*) T1 W1 in a patient who has know thyroid ophthalmopathy reveal bilateral and symmetric enlargement of all the EOMs. The inferior rectus muscles are the most involved.

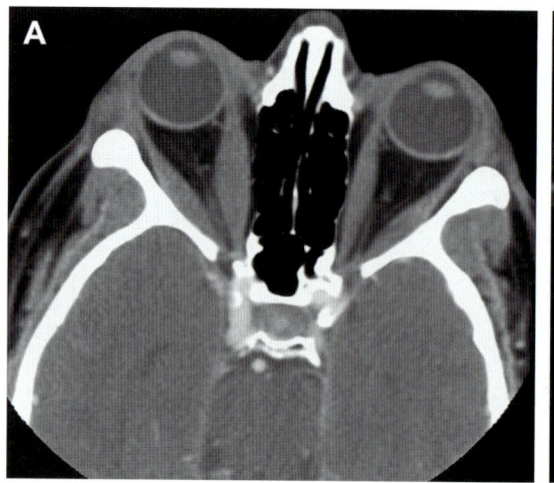
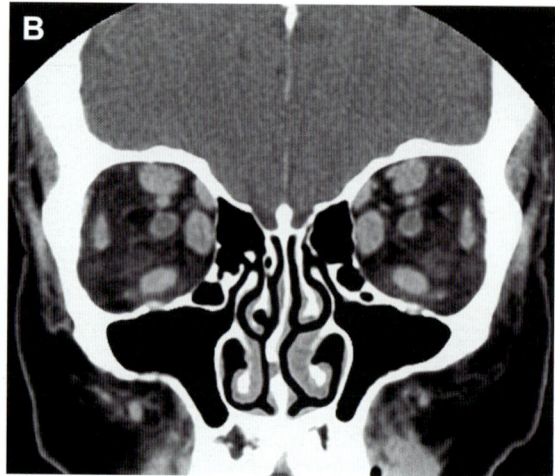

Fig. 4. Thyroid ophthalmopathy with different patterns of muscle involvement. (A) Axial CT section of the mid-orbit reveals enlargement of bilateral EOMs. Involvement is asymmetric, however, with right medial and lateral recti involved more than left side. (B) Coronal CT section at the mid-orbit shows bilateral and symmetric involvement of the EOMs. Also note the increased density and stranding of the retro-ocular fat bilaterally.

vascular malformation (especially caroticocavernous sinus fistula), metastasis, lymphoproliferative disease, parasitic involvement, and rarely orbital amyloidosis. Patients who have vascular malformation (**Fig. 10**A, B) often exhibit enlargement of the superior ophthalmic vein with obvious abnormality within the cavernous sinus. Metastases, especially from the breast, can involve single or multiple EOMs (**Fig. 10**C). They show a more nodular pattern, however, and the adjacent fat may be involved. The brain parenchyma could show features of metastatic disease (see **Fig. 10**C). Orbital pseudotumor causes muscular enlargement and is most often unilateral. In these patients the muscle involvement is ill-defined and the tendon sheaths are also involved. Clinically this condition is painful compared with thyroid ophthalmopathy. Ocular lymphoma often shows involvement of the EOMs along with adjacent soft tissue involvement. Rarely parasitic diseases, such as cysticercosis and trichinosis, can involve the EOM and present with diplopia.[37] Images often reveal a well-defined parasitic larva and involvement is usually restricted to a single muscle.

TREATMENT

Although the therapy for hyperthyroidism associated with Graves disease is fairly successful, the current treatment options for the ophthalmologic

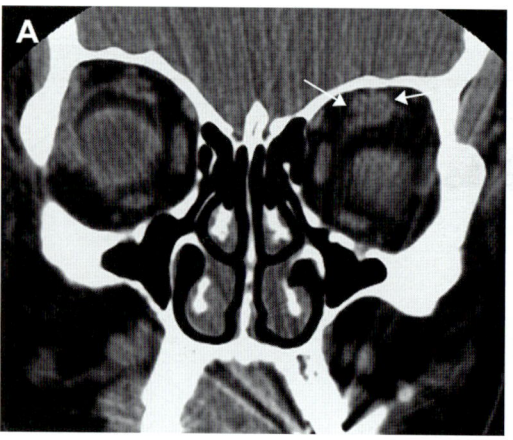
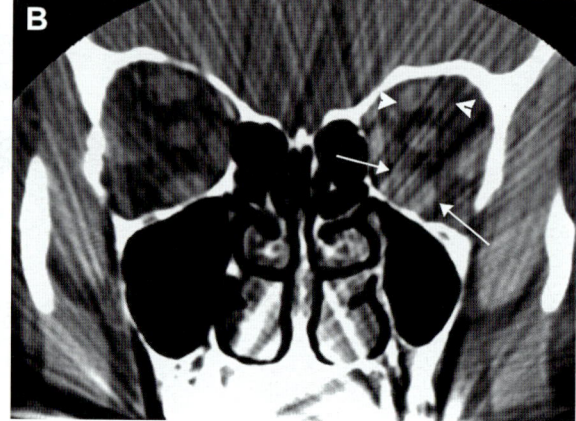

Fig. 5. Thyroid ophthalmopathy with progressive muscle involvement. (A) Coronal CT section through the orbit in a patient who has early thyroid ophthalmopathy reveals enlargement of the left superior muscle complex (arrows). (B) Follow-up CT 5 months later showed interval decrease in swelling of the superior muscles (arrowheads) but there was a new enlargement of the left inferior rectus muscle (arrows).

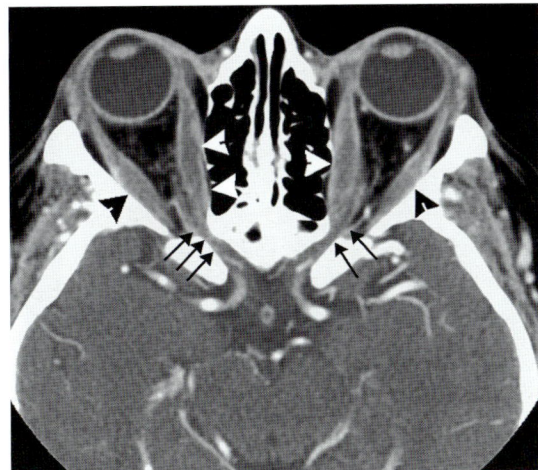

Fig. 6. Thyroid ophthalmopathy with optic nerve compression. Axial CT section of the mid-orbit in a patient who has severe enlargement of the EOMs reveals enlarged medial and lateral rectus muscles (*arrowheads*). There is loss of normal fat at the level of orbital apex (*arrows*) and resultant compression of the optic nerves bilaterally.

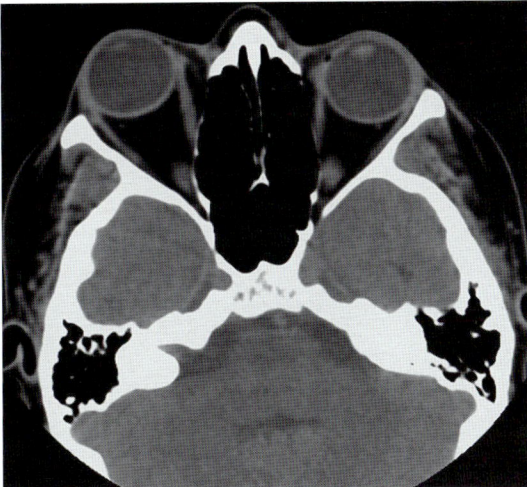

Fig. 7. Thyroid ophthalmopathy with bilateral retro-ocular fat expansion and proptosis. Axial CT section through the mid-orbit reveals bilateral (right more than left) exophthalmos secondary to retro-ocular fat expansion. There was no significant EOM enlargement.

manifestations have numerous shortcomings and are frustrating at times for the treating physician. The treatments are mostly supportive, addressing primarily the symptoms of the disease and not its causes. Most patients who have TO have external eye complaints that are self-limited and usually managed with overnight head elevation, lubrication, and topical therapies.[3] Prisms in glasses may reduce diplopia. Patients who develop severe orbital inflammation, proptosis, diplopia, and compressive optic neuropathies require more aggressive therapy. Many ophthalmologists use systemic steroids, either oral or intravenous, for short-term control of the disease. Most patients show some response to the steroids, but high doses are often required.[3,9] A subset of patients either do not respond adequately or have significant side effects that warrant stopping the

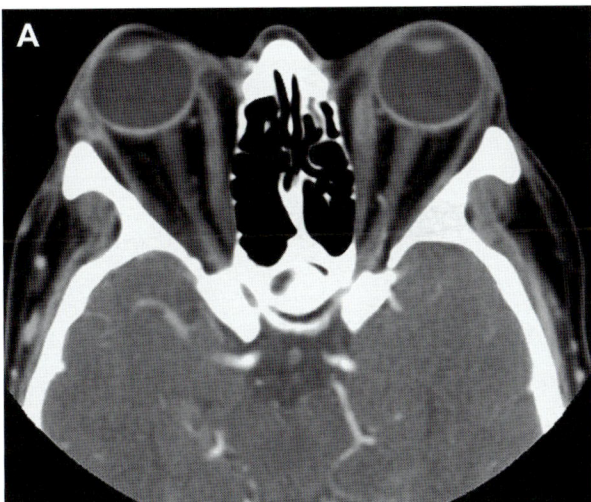
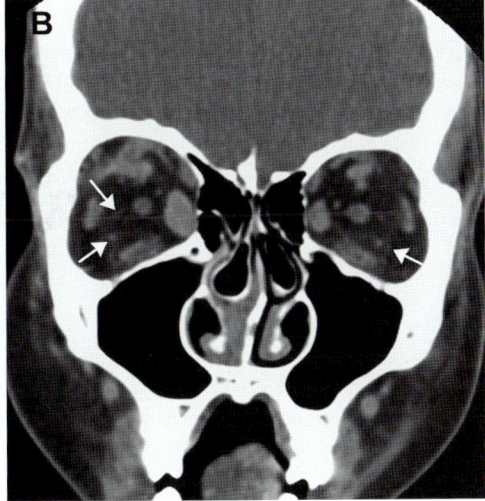

Fig. 8. Thyroid ophthalmopathy with retro-ocular fat infiltration. Axial (*A*) and coronal (*B*) CT sections at the mid-orbit level reveal expansion of the retro-ocular fat with increased density and inhomogeneous appearance of the retro-ocular fat (*arrows*). There is partial obliteration of the margins of the EOMs.

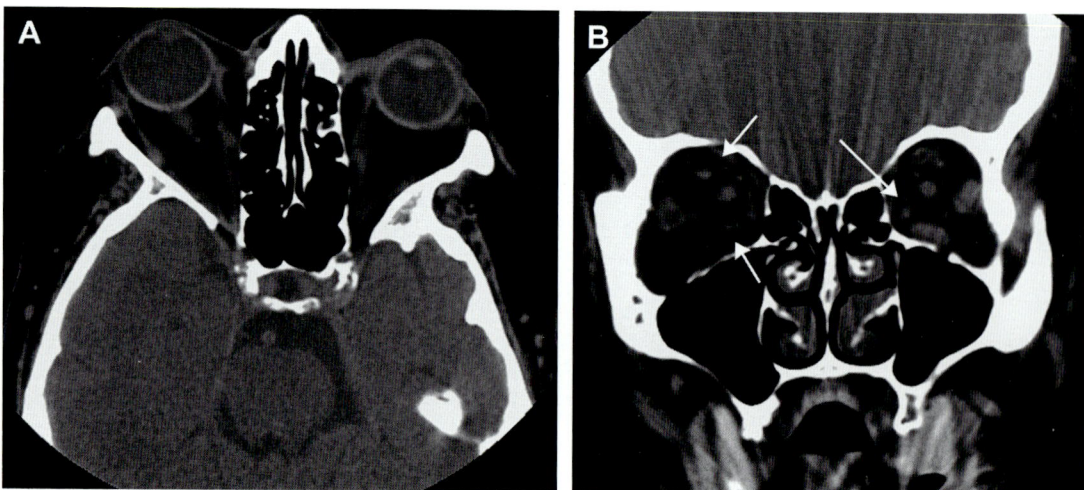

Fig. 9. Thyroid ophthalmopathy with chronic muscle changes. Axial (*A*) and coronal (*B*) CT sections through the mid-orbit in a patient who has chronic thyroid ophthalmopathy reveal atrophic-appearing EOMs with fatty replacement (*arrows*). Although the muscles show reduced swelling the retro-ocular fat expansion persists.

steroids. There are different options for treatment of these patients, but there is no definite consensus on the most appropriate treatment. Immunosuppressive medications have also been used, some with limited success, and others, such as cyclosporine, cyclophosphamide, and azathioprine, with potential benefits. Surgical orbital decompression (**Fig. 11**A–C) or external beam radiation therapy may be warranted in patients who have compressive optic neuropathies to prevent significant loss of vision. Orbital decompression surgery involves enlargement of the bony orbit and removal of hypertrophied fat. This procedure involves removal of bone from one of the four orbital walls, depending on the degree of decompression needed for an individual patient.[38]

Another important issue in the management of these patients is the control of the sequelae after the inflammation has subsided.[3] The management of diplopia and strabismus secondary to EOM inflammation or fibrosis is often a major concern of these patients and may require surgical correction.

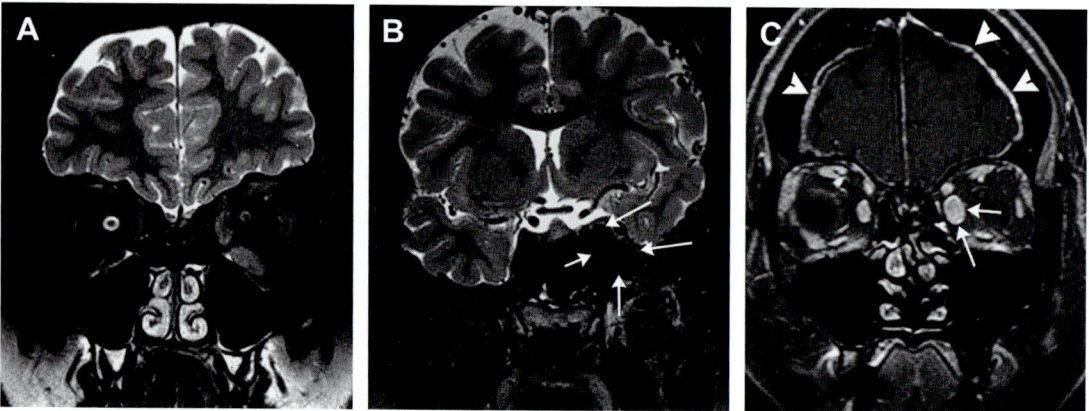

Fig. 10. Differential diagnosis for thyroid ophthalmopathy. (*A, B*) Patient who has left cavernous arteriovenous fistula. Coronal T2 WI MR imaging at mid-orbit and optic chiasm level reveals enlargement of the left EOMs, similar to thyroid ophthalmopathy. The patient has a large left cavernous arteriovenous fistula (*arrows*) and changes of venous hypertension in the left orbit. (*C*) Metastasis from breast carcinoma. Coronal contrast-enhanced T1 WI at mid-orbit level reveals enlargement of the left medial rectus muscle (*arrows*), which in this patient who has breast cancer is suggestive of metastatic lesion. Note diffuse pachymeningeal involvement (*arrowheads*).

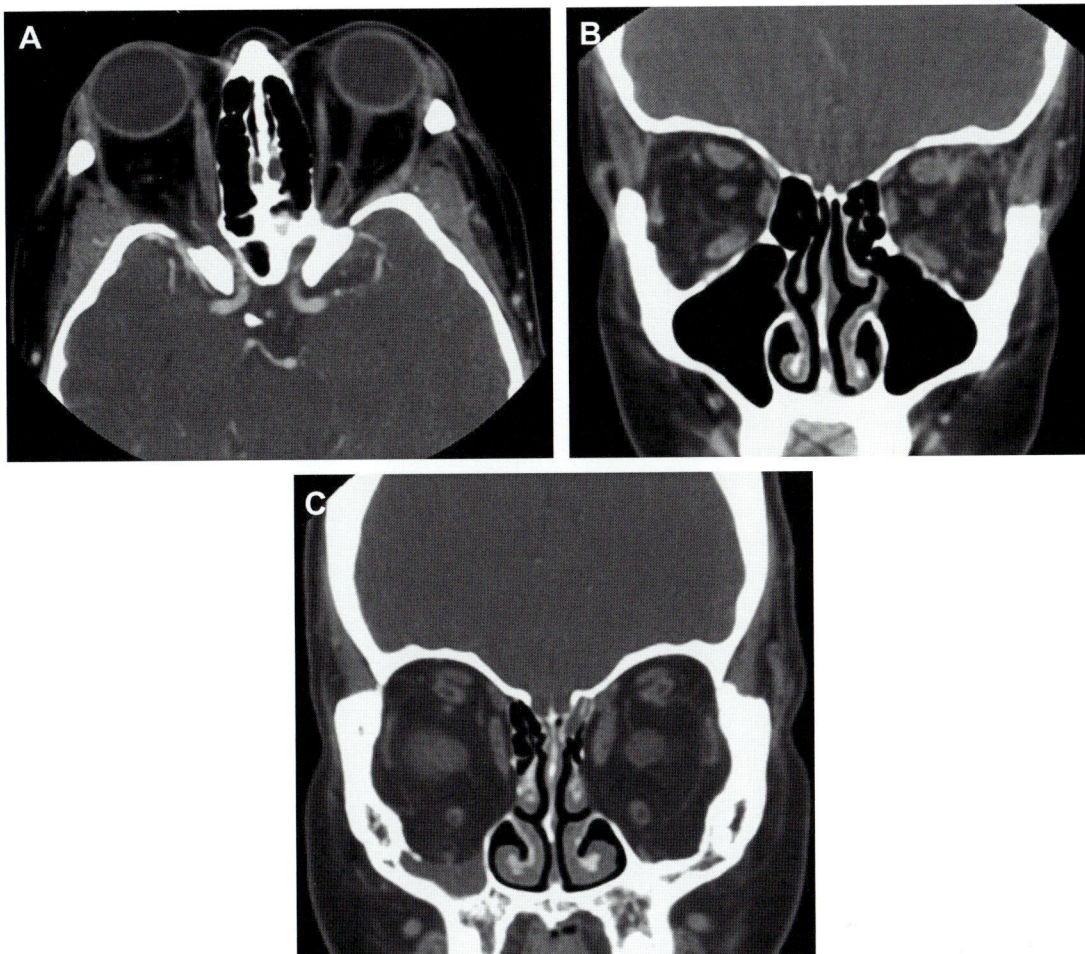

Fig. 11. Thyroid ophthalmopathy with orbital decompression. CT sections of two patients who had surgical decompression for thyroid ophthalmopathy. (A, B) Axial and coronal CT sections at mid-orbit level show removal of anterior margin of the lateral walls of the orbits. Note the lateral bowing of the lateral rectus muscles as a result of decompression. (C) Coronal CT section in another patient reveals inferior orbital decompression with displacement of the orbital fat and inferior rectus muscles.

In the patient who has complex disease, it is often recommended that orbital decompression be performed before proceeding to EOM surgery. Eyelid surgery is often deferred until both of these other procedures are done.[3]

REFERENCES

1. Halperin EC, Quaranta B. The eponymy of exophthalmos associated with thyroid disease. In: Dutton JJ, Hail BG, editors. Thyroid eye disease. New York: Marcel Dekker; 2002. p. 3–8.
2. Poster MF. Thyroid eponymy. N Engl J Med 1973; 288:422.
3. Haik BG, Calzada JI. Introduction to thyroid eye disease. In: Dutton JJ, Hail BG, editors. Thyroid eye disease. New York: Marcel Dekker; 2002. p. 1–2.
4. Ingbar SH, Woeber KA. The thyroid. In: Williams RH, editor. Textbook of endocrinology. 6th edition. Philadelphia: WB Saunders; 1981. p. 1980–1.
5. Dallow RL. Evaluation of unilateral exophthalmos with ultrasonography: analysis of 258 consecutive cases. Laryngoscope 1975;85:1905–19.
6. Grove AS. Evaluation of exophthalmos. N Engl J Med 1975;292:1005–13.
7. Hay ID. Clinical presentations of Graves's ophthalmopathy. In: Gorman CA, Waller RR, Dryer JA, editors. The eye and orbit in thyroid disease. New York: Raven Press; 1984. p. 1984–5.
8. Gorman CA. Temporal relationship between the onset of Graves's ophthalmopathy and diagnosis of thyrotoxicosis. Mayo Clin Proc 1983;58:515–9.
9. Weber AL, Dallow RL, Sabates NR. Graves' disease of the orbit. Neuroimaging Clin N Am 1996;6:61–72.

10. Prummel MF, Koornneef L, Mourits M, et al. Introduction to Graves' ophthalmopathy. In: Prummel MF, editor. Recent developments in Graves' ophthalmopathy. Norwell (MA): Kluwer Academic Publishers; 2000. p. 1–14.
11. Rundle FF, Finlay-Jones LR, Noad KB. Malignant exophthalmos: a quantitative analysis of the orbital tissues. Australas Ann Med 1953;2:1–8.
12. Ven der Gaag R, Schmidt ED, Zonneveld FW, et al. Orbital pathology in thyroid-associated ophthalmopathy. Orbit 1996;15:109–17.
13. Pappa A, Jackson P, Stone J, et al. An ultrastructural and systemic analysis of glycosaminoglycans in thyroid-associated ophthalmopathy. Eye 1998;12:237–44.
14. Hufnagel TJ, Hickey WF, Cobbs WH, et al. Immunohistochemical and ultrastructural studies on the exenterated orbital tissues of a patient with Graves' disease. Ophthalmology 1984;91:1411–9.
15. Naffziger HC. Progressive exophthalmos following thyroidectomy; its pathology and treatment. Ann Surg 1931;94:582–6.
16. Kroll AJ, Kuwabara T. Dysthyroid ocular myopathy: anatomy, histology and electron microscopy. Arch Ophthalmol 1966;76:244–57.
17. Mengistu M, Lukes YG, Nagy EV, et al. TSH receptor expression in retroocular fibroblasts. J Endocrinol Invest 1994;17:434–41.
18. Hatton MP, Rubin PAD. The pathophysiology of thyroid-associated ophthalmopathy. Ophthalmol Clin North Am 2002;15:113–9.
19. Wilson FM. Fundamentals and principles of ophthalmology. Basic and clinical science course. San Francisco (CA): American Academy of Ophthalmology; 1991–1992.
20. Heufelder AE, Weetman AP, Ludgate M, et al. Pathogenesis of Graves' ophthalmopathy. In: Prummel MF, editor. Recent developments in Graves' ophthalmopathy. Norwell (MA): Kluwer Academic Publishers; 2000. p. 15–37.
21. Jacobson DL, Gange SJ, Rose NR, et al. Epidemiology and estimated population burden of selected autoimmune disease in the United States. Clin Immunol Immunopathol 1997;84:223–43.
22. Werner SC. Modification of the classification of the eye changes of Graves' disease: recommendations of the ad hoc committee of the American Thyroid Association. J Clin Endocrinol Metab 1977;44:203–4.
23. Eden KC, Trotter WR. Lid-retraction in toxic diffuse goiter. Lancet 1942;2:386–7.
24. Noh JY, Makamura Y, Ito K, et al. Sympathetic overactivity of intraocular muscles evaluated by accommodation in patients with hyperthyroidism. Thyroid 1996;4:289–93.
25. Werner SC. The severe eye changes of Graves' disease. JAMA 1961;177:81–5.
26. Dobyns BM. Present concepts of the pathologic physiology of exophthalmos. J Clin Endocrinol Metab 1950;10:1202–30.
27. Koornneef L, Schmidt ED, Van der Gaag R. The orbit: structure, autoantigens and pathology. In: Wall J, How J, editors. Graves' ophthalmopathy. Oxford (UK): Blackwell Scientific Publications; 1990. p. 1–16.
28. Rundle FF, Pochin EE. The orbital tissues in thyrotoxicosis: a quantitative analysis relating to exophthalmos. Clin Sci 1944;5:51–74.
29. Tanner V, Tregear SJ, Ripley LG, et al. Automated achromatic contrast and chromatic discrimination sensitivity testing in dysthyroid optic neuropathy. Eye 1995;9:352–7.
30. Dolman PJ, Rootman J. VISA classification for Graves orbitopathy. Ophthal Plast Reconstr Surg 2006;22:319–24.
31. Mafee MF, Miller MT. Computed tomography scanning in the evaluation of ocular motility disorders. In: Gonzalez CF, Becker MH, Flanagan JC, editors. Diagnostic imaging in ophthalmology. New York: Springer-Verlag; 1985. p. 39–54.
32. Rubin RM, Sadun AA. Ocular myopathies. In: Yanoff M, Duker JS, editors. Ophthalmology. St. Louis: CV Mosby; 1999. p. 11.18.1–11.18.8.
33. Enzmann D, Marshall WH, Rosenthal AR. Computed tomography in Graves' ophthalmopathy. Radiology 1976;118:615–20.
34. Rootman J, editor. Diseases of the orbit. Philadelphia: JB Lippincott; 1988.
35. Barrett L, Glatt HJ, Burde RM, et al. Optic nerve dysfunction in thyroid eye disease. Radiology 1988;167:503–7.
36. Feldon SE, Weiner JM. Clinical significance of extraocular muscle volume in Graves' ophthalmopathy. Arch Ophthalmol 1982;100:1266–9.
37. Ursekar MA, Dastur DK, Manghani DK, et al. Isolated cyticercal infestation of extraocular muscles: CT and MR findings. AJNR Am J Neuroradiol 1998;19:109–13.
38. Goldberg RA. The evolving paradigm of orbital decompression. Arch Ophthalmol 1998;166:95–6.

Parathyroid Imaging

Saeed Fakhran, MD[a], Barton F. Branstetter, IV, MD[a,b], Daniel A. Pryma, MD[c,]*

KEYWORDS
- Parathyroid Glands • Hyperparathyroidism
- Parathyroid Adenoma • Parathyroid Carcinoma

EMBRYOLOGY AND ANATOMY

The parathyroid glands develop at 6 weeks of fetal life and migrate caudally at 8 weeks. The paired superior parathyroid glands derive, along with the thyroid gland, from the dorsal portions of the fourth branchial pouch. The superior parathyroid glands tend to be consistent in position, posterior and lateral to the upper pole of the thyroid, at the level of the cricoid cartilage, along the inferior thyroid artery and recurrent laryngeal nerve. The inferior parathyroid glands, along with the thymus, develop from the third branchial pouch and migrate caudally to rest inferior to the relatively less mobile superior parathyroid glands. Occasionally the inferior parathyroid glands migrate to the level of the aortic arch, or in rare circumstances, fail to migrate and remain in the high neck.[1–4]

The parathyroid glands are usually located between the posterior border of the thyroid gland and its fibrous capsule, although they can be intrathyroidal also. A normal parathyroid gland has dimensions of 5 × 3 × 1 mm and weight of 30 to 40 mg. Although most patients have four parathyroid glands, approximately 5% have fewer, and 3% to 13% have supernumerary glands.[3,5,6]

PATHOLOGY
Hyperparathyroidism

Hyperparathyroidism can be primary, secondary, or tertiary. Primary hyperparathyroidism, defined as an independent focus of parathyroid hormone overproduction, has an estimated prevalence of 1:7000 in the United States. Women are affected approximately twice to three times as often as men. Diagnosis is based on elevated calcium and parathyroid hormone levels and clinical symptoms consist of renal calculi, gastric ulcers, bone cysts, and mental depression. In the vast majority of patients (approximately 85%), a single parathyroid adenoma is the cause of disease (**Fig. 1**); the remaining causes include diffuse hyperplasia (10%), multiple adenomas (4%), or rarely parathyroid carcinoma or cysts.[7–9]

Secondary hyperparathyroidism occurs because of hyperplasia of the parathyroid glands following long-term hyperstimulation and parathyroid hormone release. In contrast to primary hyperparathyroidism, elevated parathyroid hormone levels do not result in hypercalcemia. Classically this has been ascribed to most patients who have secondary hyperparathyroidism suffering from chronic renal failure and therefore having an underlying hypocalcemic state, although this has not been fully elucidated. Rarer causes of secondary hyperparathyroidism include diminished calcitriol levels, resistance to parathyroid hormone by skeletal tissue, rickets, and malabsorption syndromes.[10,11]

Following long-term hyperstimulation, the parathyroid glands start to function autonomously and produce high levels of parathyroid hormone, despite correction of underlying chronic hypocalcemia. Tertiary hyperparathyroidism refers to the subsequent hypercalcemia produced by this autonomous parathyroid function.[10,11]

---

[a] Department of Radiology, University of Pittsburgh, 200 Lothrop Street, PUH Room D132, Pittsburgh, PA 15213, USA
[b] Department of Otolaryngology, University of Pittsburgh, 200 Lothrop Street, PUH Room D132, Pittsburgh, PA 15213, USA
[c] Division of Nuclear Medicine and Clinical Molecular Imaging, Department of Radiology, University of Pennsylvania, Donner 110, 3400 Spruce Street, Philadelphia, PA 19104, USA
* Corresponding author.
E-mail address: Daniel.Pryma@uphs.upenn.edu (D.A. Pryma).

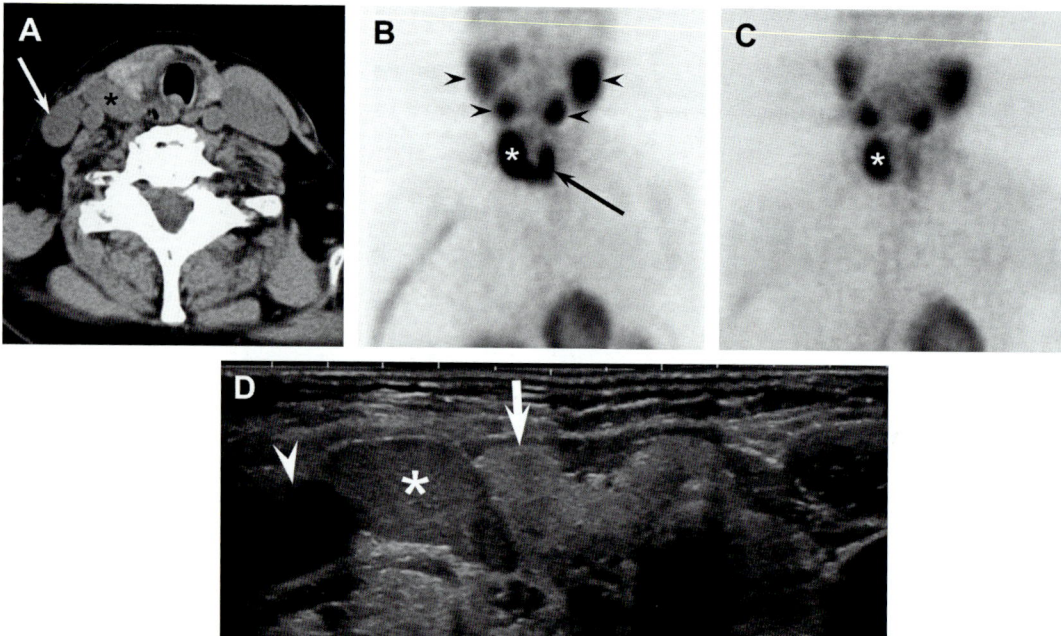

Fig. 1. Parathyroid adenoma. (A) Unenhanced CT shows an oval mass (*) uniformly isodense to vessels that might be confused with the internal jugular vein, except that the vein is visible laterally (arrow). (B) Early three-dimensional sestamibi image in frontal projection shows uptake in the mass (*) and physiologic uptake in the salivary glands (arrowheads) and thyroid gland (arrow). (C) Late sestamibi image shows retention of radiotracer in the adenoma (*), with washout (absence) of radiotracer in the thyroid gland. The salivary glands normally retain radiotracer on late images. (D) Sonographic image in transverse plane shows the adenoma (*) with uniform intermediate echogenicity, situated between the right thyroid lobe (arrow) and the carotid artery (arrrowhead).

Multiple Endocrine Neoplasia

Multiple endocrine neoplasia (MEN) is a hereditary syndrome characterized by abnormal function of two or more endocrine organs. MEN1 is characterized by primary hyperparathyroidism, pancreatic endocrine tumors, and anterior pituitary gland neoplasms, whereas MEN2A is characterized by pheochromocytomas, medullary thyroid carcinoma, and hyperparathyroidism. In both cases the hyperparathyroidism is multiglandular; however, in MEN1 it is characterized by an asynchronous and steadily progressive course, whereas in MEN2A it has a later onset and less severe effects at clinical evaluation, with lower morbidity.[3,12–15]

Parathyroid Cysts

There are two types of parathyroid cysts. The first is a purely cystic parathyroid lesion, attributable to embryologic remnants of the third or fourth branchial pouches or enlargement of microcysts within the parathyroid because of colloid retention (Fig. 2). The second type refers to cystic necrosis or degeneration of parathyroid adenomas. Both entities can cause hypercalcemia because of high parathyroid hormone level in the cyst fluid.[3,6,16]

Parathyroid Carcinoma

Carcinoma occurs in 0.5% to 1.0% of patients who have primary hyperparathyroidism. It is usually indistinguishable from benign adenoma on clinical evaluation and imaging (Fig. 3). It can be suggested by a palpable neck mass on examination or demonstration of invasion of adjacent structures on imaging, however. Classically, parathyroid carcinomas are said to be slow growing with distant metastasis occurring late in the course of the disease.[6,16]

Parathyromatosis

Parathyromatosis is a rare condition characterized by findings of multiple rests of hyperfunctioning parathyroid tissue in the neck and mediastinum with resultant persistent or recurrent hyperparathyroidism (Fig. 4). It has been associated with MEN1, spillage of hypercellular parathyroid tissue during surgical exploration of the neck, or hyperfunctioning parathyroid rests left behind during ontogenesis.[17,18] Importantly, ultrasound-guided fine

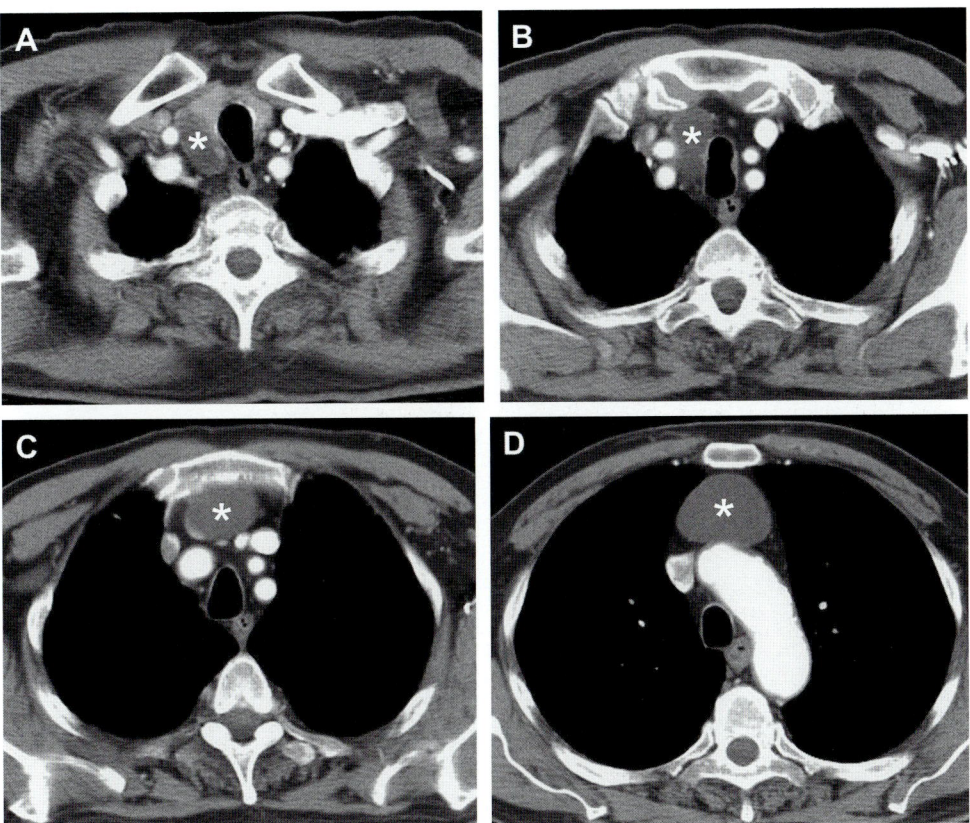

Fig. 2. Parathyroid cyst. Enhanced CT images through the lower neck and chest reveal a fluid-density mass (asterisks) that extends from the right tracheoesophageal groove (*A*), into the paratracheal superior mediastinum (*B*), then into the substernal region (*C*), and anterior to the aortic arch (*D*). Other cystic neck masses, such as thymic cyst or lymphangioma, might have similar extent and appearance.

needle aspiration does not seem to predispose patients to development of parathyromatosis.[19]

PARATHYROID IMAGING

Several modalities can be used to image the parathyroid gland. Because hyperparathyroidism caused by a solitary parathyroid adenoma is by far the most common form of parathyroid pathology, imaging is often geared toward accurate preoperative identification of the offending adenoma. Accurate preoperative identification of a parathyroid adenoma allows for directed parathyroid surgery, which is as effective as traditional bilateral neck exploration, but is associated with reduced surgical time, reduced hospital stay, improved cosmetic result, use of local rather than general anesthesia, and no risk for permanent hypoparathyroidism.[9,20–24] This identification can be accomplished with neck ultrasound, ^{99m}Tc sestamibi scintigraphy, or, ideally, a combination of both. CT and MR imaging are primarily used to further evaluate suspected cases of parathyroid carcinoma and parathyroid cysts, although they can also be used to aid in diagnosis in select cases of hyperparathyroidism.[25]

Ultrasound

Technique
Imaging should be performed with 10-MHz or higher linear array transducers to provide optimal gray-scale and color Doppler imaging. The patient is examined in the supine position with the neck slightly extended, identical to the position used to scan the thyroid gland. Rotation of the neck away from the side being examined and asking the patient to swallow may aide in locating enlarged parathyroid glands. Scanning is performed in the transverse and longitudinal planes with attention focused posterior and inferior to the thyroid gland, medial to the carotid artery and jugular vein, and along the tracheoesophageal groove. If necessary the transducer can be angled to increase visualization inferiorly along the trachea and into the superior mediastinum or behind the clavicle. Graded compression may also aid

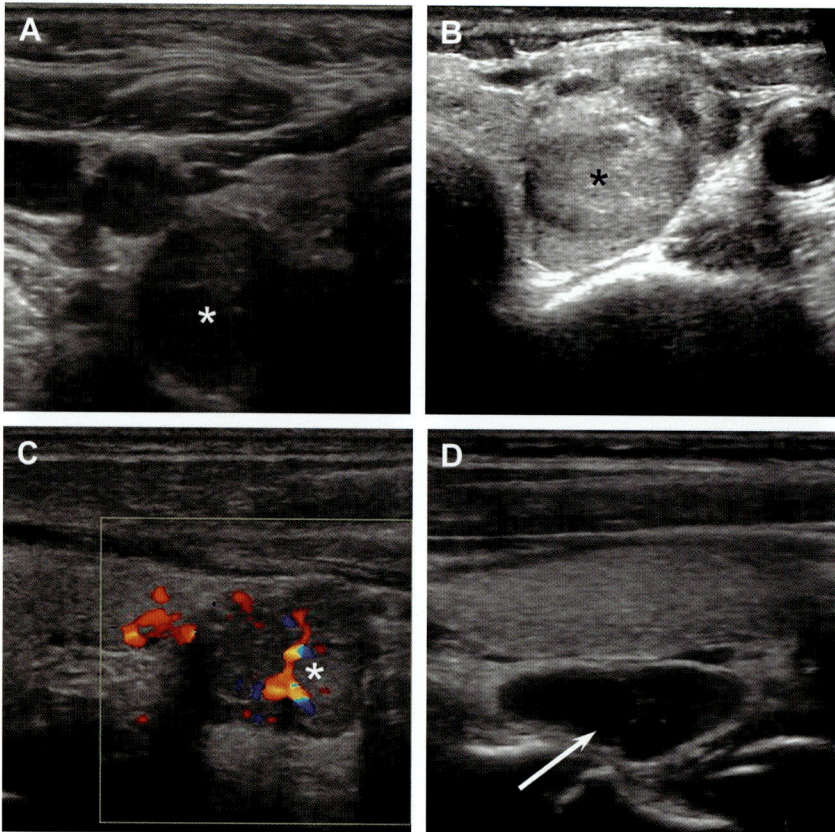

Fig. 3. Parathyroid carcinoma. Sonographic images from three patients who had parathyroid carcinoma (*A–C*) and one patient who had parathyroid adenoma (*D*). There are no reliable distinguishing characteristics for the carcinomas (*asterisks*). They may be of low (*A*) or high (*B*) echogenicity, and may have Doppler flow (*C*) similar to that of an adenoma. Adenomas (*arrow*) may be more compressible and thus appear to be oriented more longitudinally on compressed views (*D*), but this is not a reliable sign.

in differentiating a relatively incompressible gland from surrounding soft tissue.[1] Color Doppler sonography should be performed on all suspected adenomas because vascularity is important to the sonographic diagnosis (**Fig. 5**).

Interpretation

The normal parathyroid gland is typically not visualized because of its deep location and small size. Parathyroid adenomas larger than 1 cm should be visible on ultrasound. Parathyroid adenomas are usually ovoid, well-marginated, solid lesions. As opposed to cervical lymph nodes, with which adenomas may be confused, adenomas have a homogeneously hypoechoic internal echotexture and lack a central echogenic hilum. Hypoechogenicity may be related to the marked, compact cellularity of parathyroid adenomas that is evident on pathologic examination.[1] It is important for the sonographer to continue searching for other abnormal glands even when one is already discovered. In cases in which multiple hyperplastic glands are present, each individual gland will likely appear similar to an adenoma, and ultrasound evaluation is unable to differentiate multiple adenomas from parathyroid hyperplasia.

Parathyroid adenomas are typically highly vascular lesions and this vascularity is reflected on color Doppler sonography. Adenomas have a peripheral vascular arc arising from a feeding vessel, often a branch of the inferior thyroidal artery, which partially encircles the adenoma. This structure is contradistinctive from lymph nodes, which are typically supplied by small hilar vessels. This polar vascularity may be helpful in identifying adenomas in confusing or difficult cases; however, vascularity is variable and cannot be relied on alone.[6]

Parathyroid carcinomas are difficult to distinguish from parathyroid adenomas on the basis of sonography alone. Keeping in mind that parathyroid carcinoma accounts for less than 1% of parathyroid abnormalities, one may suspect carcinoma if an unusually large adenoma with a thick

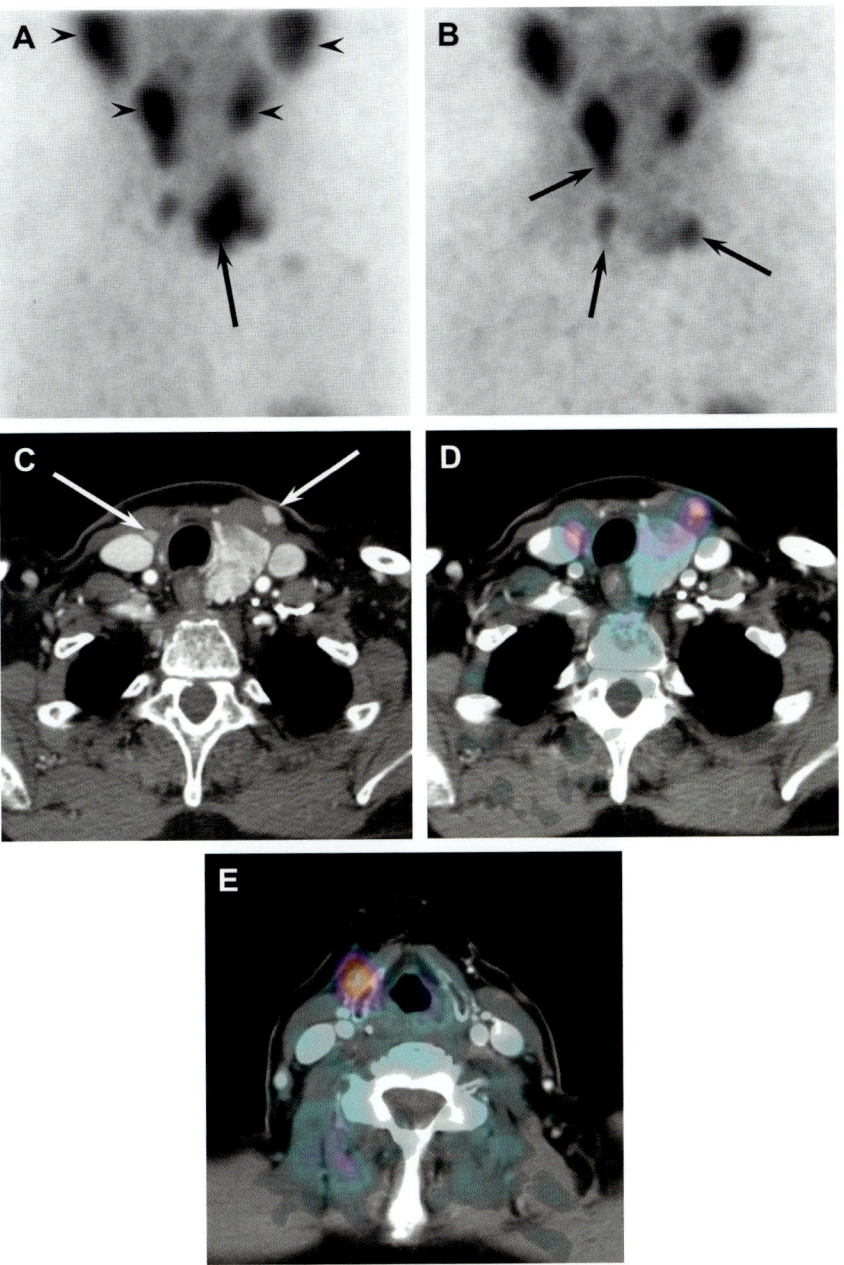

Fig. 4. Parathyromatosis. (A) Early sestamibi image shows physiologic uptake in the thyroid gland (arrow) and salivary glands (arrowheads), and several other foci scattered through the neck. (B) Late sestamibi image confirms that many of these additional foci (arrows) are rests of hyperfunctioning parathyroid tissue. (C) Axial contrast-enhanced CT image shows multiple nonspecific briskly enhancing nodules (arrows), which correspond to the increased sestamibi uptake on fused SPECT-CT (D and E).

capsule or markedly increased vascularity is seen. Carcinomas may also demonstrate cystic degeneration, calcification, or increased internal heterogeneity.[6,16] In advanced cases, local tissue invasion and regional lymphadenopathy may be identified.

Parathyroid cysts have the same sonographic appearance as cysts seen elsewhere in the body (Fig. 6). These lesions occur inferior to the inferior thyroid pole margin in 95% of cases and 65% involve the inferior parathyroid glands.[6]

Pitfalls

Using the above techniques recent studies report a sensitivity ranging from 27% to 97% with most values clustering around 70% (range 27%–97%

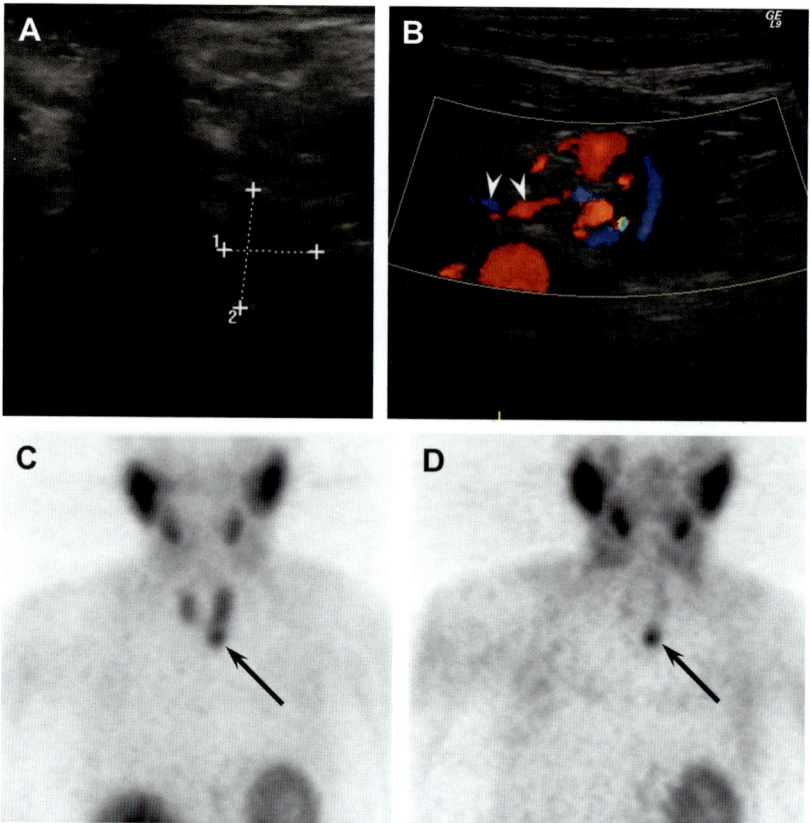

Fig. 5. Parathyroid adenoma. (*A*) Transverse sonographic image through the thyroid bed shows a uniformly hypoechoic mass posterior to the left thyroid lobe. (*B*) Doppler sonography shows robust vascularity within the mass and a central feeding vessel (*arrowheads*). (*C*) Early sestamibi image shows a focus of uptake (*arrow*) at the inferior tip of the left thyroid lobe, corresponding to the sonographic abnormality. (*D*) Late sestamibi image shows persistent uptake, differentiating this parathyroid adenoma from thyroid pathology.

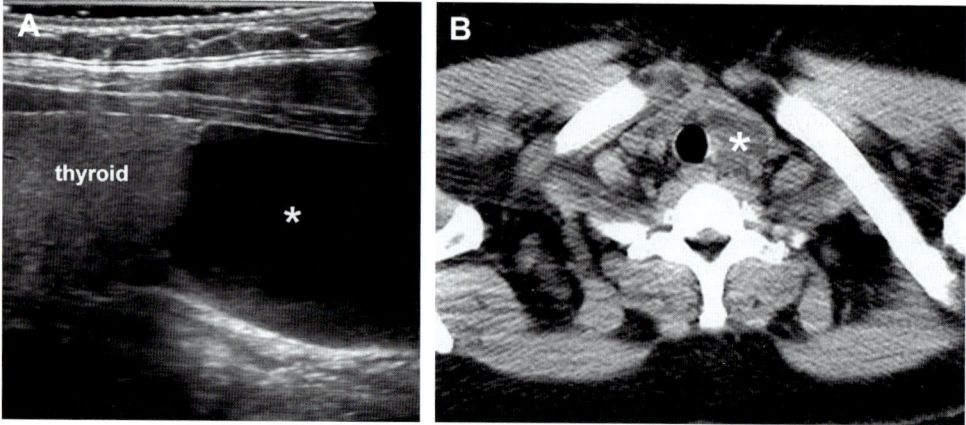

Fig. 6. Parathyroid cyst. (*A*) Longitudinal sonographic image shows an anechoic mass (*) inferior to the left thyroid lobe. (*B*) Axial CT image shows a corresponding low-density mass immediately posterior to the inferior aspect of the left thyroid lobe. The CT cannot distinguish cyst from solid mass, and cannot distinguish parathyroid from thyroid pathology. Tissue sampling is usually necessary for diagnosis.

for single-gland disease, 50%–90% for carcinoma, 40%–50% for hyperplasia).[8,26] In a recent meta-analysis the sensitivity for ultrasound was 79% for detecting solitary adenoma, 16% for detecting double adenomas, 35% for hyperplasia, and 100% for carcinoma.[8,27] The wide range of sensitivities is reflective of the difficulties inherent to this examination. Major pitfalls of ultrasound relate to errors of detection and characterization. It is often difficult for inexperienced (and even experienced) sonographers to detect ectopic or intrathyroid nodules. Glands in retroesophageal and mediastinal locations or within the carotid sheath can be especially difficult to detect. Ultrasound is of limited value in cases of adenomas in a deep paratracheal, paraesophageal, and mediastinal location, because these lesions are inaccessible to the ultrasound beam.[9]

The presence of concomitant thyroid disease can add further complexity and confusion to an already difficult examination. Intrathyroidal adenomas can often mimic thyroid nodules, whereas exophytic thyroid nodules may mimic parathyroid adenomas. In patients who have underlying inflammatory disorders of the thyroid gland, such as Hashimoto thyroiditis, adenomas can be especially difficult to detect.[6,22,26] These patients often have multiple prominent central compartment lymph nodes that may mask or mimic parathyroid adenomas.

A recent analysis suggests that false-negative ultrasound images were related to characterization errors at least as often, if not more often, than errors of detection, and that size is not necessarily a limiting factor. In that study 62% of undetected nodules were greater than 2 cm in maximum diameter, whereas 75% of detected nodules were less than 2 cm in maximum diameter.[26] Mischaracterized nodules included intrathyroidal nodules, nodules located beneath the carotid sheath, retrothyroidal nodules associated with large goiters, and nodules in patients who had chronic autoimmune thyroiditis.

The importance of well-trained and experienced operators in performing and interpreting this difficult examination cannot be overstated. For best results, performance and interpretation of parathyroid ultrasound must be a major part of a practice, not an examination performed sporadically.

Nuclear Medicine

Technique
There are many available techniques for nuclear medicine parathyroid imaging. Nuclear medicine approaches to imaging abnormal parathyroid glands rely on different radiotracer uptake patterns and kinetics between the thyroid gland, the normal parathyroid gland, and the abnormal parathyroid gland. For example, radioiodine is organified by the thyroid gland, whereas blood flow tracers such as ^{201}thallous chloride and ^{99m}Tc sestamibi identify both thyroid and enlarged parathyroid glands. These different uptake patterns can therefore be exploited with subtraction of a radioiodine image from a ^{99m}Tc sestamibi image to reveal abnormal parathyroid glands. Similarly ^{99m}Tc pertechnetate may be used instead of radioiodine. Subtraction imaging is complicated by patient motion, however, and essentially limited to planar imaging.

To take advantage of the altered tracer kinetics of abnormal parathyroid glands, dual time point imaging using either ^{201}thallous chloride or ^{99m}Tc sestamibi can be performed.[28] Typically imaging is performed within 10 minutes after tracer administration and repeated at 2 to 3 hours after tracer administration. Abnormal parathyroid glands are characterized by decreased clearance of tracer over time compared with normal parathyroid or thyroid glands.[3] Imaging can be performed using planar, single photon emission computed tomography (SPECT), SPECT-CT, or a combination of the techniques.[29]

At our center, we position the patient in the supine position with the neck extended. A dual-headed gamma camera is positioned centered on the base of the neck and extending from the skull base to the midchest. The patient is injected intravenously with approximately 925 MBq (25 mCi) ^{99m}Tc sestamibi. After a 10-minute delay, SPECT imaging is initiated. SPECT image acquisition is done with a 128 × 128 matrix size with 128 frames at 30 seconds per frame. Planar images are not routinely acquired. After a 3-hour delay from injection, the patient is repositioned under the camera making every effort to duplicate the positioning from the initial image set and SPECT imaging is repeated using the same parameters. Images are reconstructed into transverse, sagittal, coronal, and maximum intensity projection image sets using filtered back projection.

Interpretation
To optimize localization of abnormal parathyroid glands, SPECT imaging is preferred because parathyroid glands can be difficult to discriminate from the thyroid gland, particularly on early imaging, resulting in decreased sensitivity.[29] For SPECT interpretation, early and late image sets should be reviewed side-by-side. The early images are reviewed for tracer activity outside the normal contours of the thyroid gland. Furthermore,

a careful evaluation for ectopic glands should be undertaken, particularly in the mediastinum (Fig. 7). Any focal activity outside the thyroid on the early images that persists on the delayed images is highly suggestive of parathyroid adenoma. Focal activity outside the normal contours of the thyroid gland that do not show delayed washout on the late image set are equivocal but still concerning for parathyroid adenoma.

Pitfalls

Greatest among the difficulties in interpretations of ^{99m}Tc sestamibi scintigraphy are the lack of a parathyroid-specific radiotracer and the relatively high incidence of concurrent thyroid pathology. Because ^{99m}Tc sestamibi is not parathyroid specific, detection of abnormal parathyroid glands requires not only altered tracer kinetics in the abnormal parathyroid gland but also unaltered kinetics in the surrounding structures. Unfortunately, this scenario does not always exist. For example, we have seen many examples of pathologically unremarkable solitary parathyroid adenomas that do not display delayed washout of ^{99m}Tc sestamibi. Conversely, thyroid nodules, particularly Hürthle cell adenomas and carcinomas, can have very prominent ^{99m}Tc sestamibi with marked tracer retention on delayed imaging, mimicking a parathyroid adenoma.[30] On the other hand, a patient who has hypothyroidism caused, for example, by lymphocytic thyroiditis, may have very heterogeneous ^{99m}Tc sestamibi uptake by the thyroid gland making localization of abnormal parathyroid glands difficult. SPECT-CT, when available, can certainly simplify the localization of abnormal parathyroid glands, improving the sensitivity of ^{99m}Tc sestamibi scintigraphy.[29]

CT

Technique

Imaging is performed with the patient in supine position and the neck in slight extension. If not contraindicated, imaging should be performed following the administration of iodinated contrast. Volume of contrast used may range anywhere from 90 to 125 mL of iodinated contrast medium, administered at a rate of 2 to 2.5 mL/s. Using a single breath hold, 1.25 to 3.5 mm axial sections are obtained from the angle of the mandible through the aortic root, ensuring that the common locations for ectopic parathyroid adenomas and local extension of parathyroid carcinoma are included.

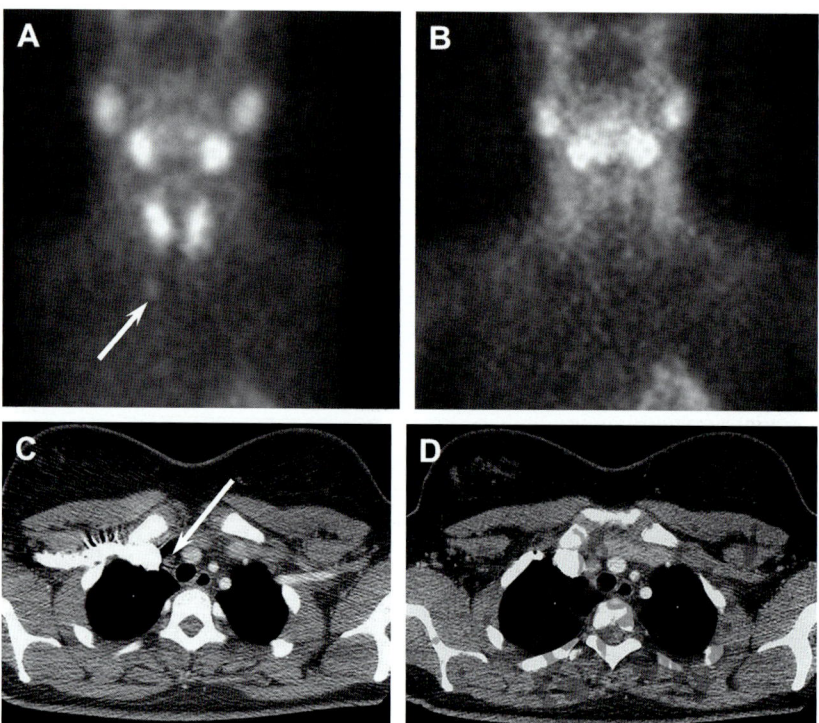

Fig. 7. Ectopic parathyroid adenoma. (*A*) Early sestamibi scan shows a focus of uptake (*arrow*) in the right superior mediastinum. (*B*) Late image shows no definite persistence. (*C*) Contrast-enhanced CT, compromised by streak artifact from undiluted contrast, shows an equivocal mass (*arrow*) in the region of sestamibi uptake. (*D*) Fused CT and sestamibi SPECT confirms correspondence of CT and nuclear medicine abnormalities.

Images may be reconstructed in the coronal, sagittal, and oblique planes and depending on radiologist preference, image interpretation in a cine loop may be helpful.

A relatively new phenomenon is the use of four-dimensional CT (4D-CT) as the primary modality in the diagnosis of primary hyperparathyroidism. 4D-CT is similar in technique to CT angiography; typically precontrast, postcontrast, and delayed images are obtained from the angle of the mandible to the upper mediastinum using 1.25-mm axial sections with 2.5-mm sagittal, coronal, and oblique reconstructions. The fourth, and added, dimension derives from changes in contrast perfusion over time.[31]

Interpretation

In most medical centers, CT is used as adjuvant imaging in difficult cases of suspected parathyroid adenoma or hyperplasia—most commonly to search for ectopic parathyroid adenomas in locations not easily accessible by ultrasound (such as the deeper paraesophageal region and mediastinum), in settings in which ultrasound is unrevealing, and particularly to correlate with ^{99m}Tc sestamibi scintigraphy findings. CT is also used in cases of recurrent primary hyperparathyroidism. Ectopic parathyroid adenomas have a nonspecific imaging appearance, typically appearing as 1 to 2 cm soft tissue density nodules on noncontrast imaging, similar in appearance to a lymph node. On contrast administration, adenomas typically demonstrate rapid uptake of contrast. In the case of 4D-CT, the hyperfunctioning parathyroid gland demonstrates more rapid uptake and washout of contrast than other structures in the neck, including normal parathyroid glands.[31]

A second major use of contrast-enhanced CT is to aid in the management of de novo or, more commonly, recurrent parathyroid carcinoma. Up to 40% to 60% of patients who have parathyroid carcinoma recur in the surgical bed within 5 years, often with local nodal involvement and, less commonly, distant metastasis.[32] Accurate preoperative localization and characterization of tumor extent is crucial for effective surgical treatment.

Pitfalls

The principal difficulty inherent in CT imaging of parathyroid disease is the relatively nonspecific appearance of hyperfunctioning parathyroid glands on cross-sectional imaging. This difficulty is magnified by the relatively complex anatomy inherent to imaging of the neck and superior mediastinum and the small size of many pathologic parathyroid glands, making interpretation of these studies challenging even to experienced practitioners (**Fig. 8**). When interpreting CT of parathyroid disease, it is not only helpful but almost mandatory to have additional imaging—in the form of ultrasound or ^{99m}Tc sestamibi scintigraphy—that directs the radiologist to the most likely location of the abnormal parathyroid glands and aids in the differentiation of the parathyroid gland from nonpathologic lymph nodes, postoperative granulomas, or other benign soft tissue nodules.[25]

4D-CT is a promising new tool for the endocrinologist and the radiologist, with some studies reporting sensitivities as high as 88% for localization of hyperfunctioning parathyroid glands to one side of the neck.[31] There are significant disadvantages to this technique, however, including significantly increased expense, availability, patient radiation exposure, and a relative lack of experience and validation (especially compared with ultrasound and ^{99m}Tc sestamibi scintigraphy) that have thus far prevented its widespread use.

In cases of parathyroid carcinoma, CT is again used as part of a multi-imaging approach to aid in operative planning and optimal localization of recurrent disease. It must be realized, however, that CT is not optimal as a first-line imaging modality to evaluate recurrences in the surgical bed, with sensitivities as low as 53% in such situations.[32] CT may be used in conjunction with ^{99m}Tc sestamibi scintigraphy, however, as an adjunct for anatomic correlation, with sensitivity increasing to 67% in such situations.[32] CT is, however, optimally suited as a first-line modality in the evaluation of pulmonary, tracheoesophageal groove, and superior mediastinal metastases.

MR Imaging

Technique

Imaging is performed with the patient in a supine position and the neck in slight extension. Gadolinium-based contrast is used in all patients who do not have contraindications. Typical volume of contrast used is 13 to 16 mL. Axial, sagittal, and coronal images are obtained from the angle of the mandible through the aortic root. Optimally, an anterior neck surface coil is used for neck imaging and a torso phased array coil for mediastinal imaging. At our institution, we use a slice thickness of 3 to 5 mm with a 1-mm interslice gap. For neck imaging we use a 22-cm field of view and matrix size that varies from 256 × 192 to 320 × 224. Images are obtained with T1 and T2 weighting with fat suppression.

Interpretation

In most institutions MR imaging is used as adjunct imaging in difficult cases of suspected parathyroid

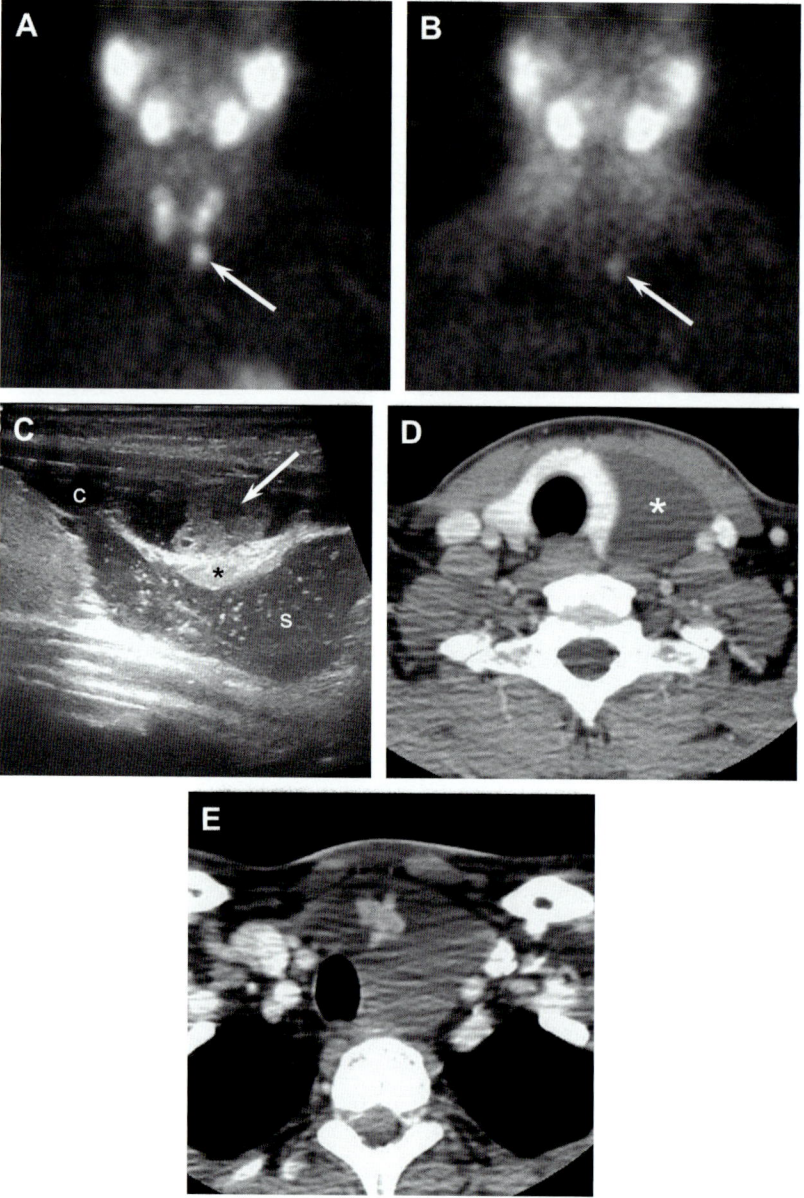

Fig. 8. Complex parathyroid adenoma/cyst. (A) Early sestamibi scan shows a small focus of uptake (arrow) below the left thyroid gland. (B) Late images show faint retention of radiotracer (arrow), suggestive of adenoma. (C) Sonography shows a complex mass with cystic (c) and heterogeneously solid (s) components, and a dense central septum (*). A central nodule (arrow) is also seen adjacent to the septum. This sonographic appearance could represent degenerated adenoma or carcinoma. (D) Contrast enhanced CT at the level of the thyroid gland shows a mass (*) of uniform low density, most consistent with parathyroid cyst. (E) CT image at the thoracic inlet shows the central nodule, but does not distinguish the cystic and solid components of the mass as well as the ultrasound does. Careful histopathologic analysis showed no evidence of carcinoma within this combined parathyroid adenoma and cyst.

adenoma or hyperplasia, often to search for ectopic parathyroid adenomas. Normal parathyroid glands may not be evident on MR imaging, whereas abnormal parathyroid glands appear as enhancing, abnormal masses in characteristic locations with increased signal intensity on T2-weighted MR imaging sequences, while being relatively isointense on T1-weighted sequences (**Fig. 9**). Unfortunately, 30% to 40% of abnormal parathyroid glands do not have these typical signal intensity characteristics. They may appear as isointense on both T1- and T2-weighted sequences

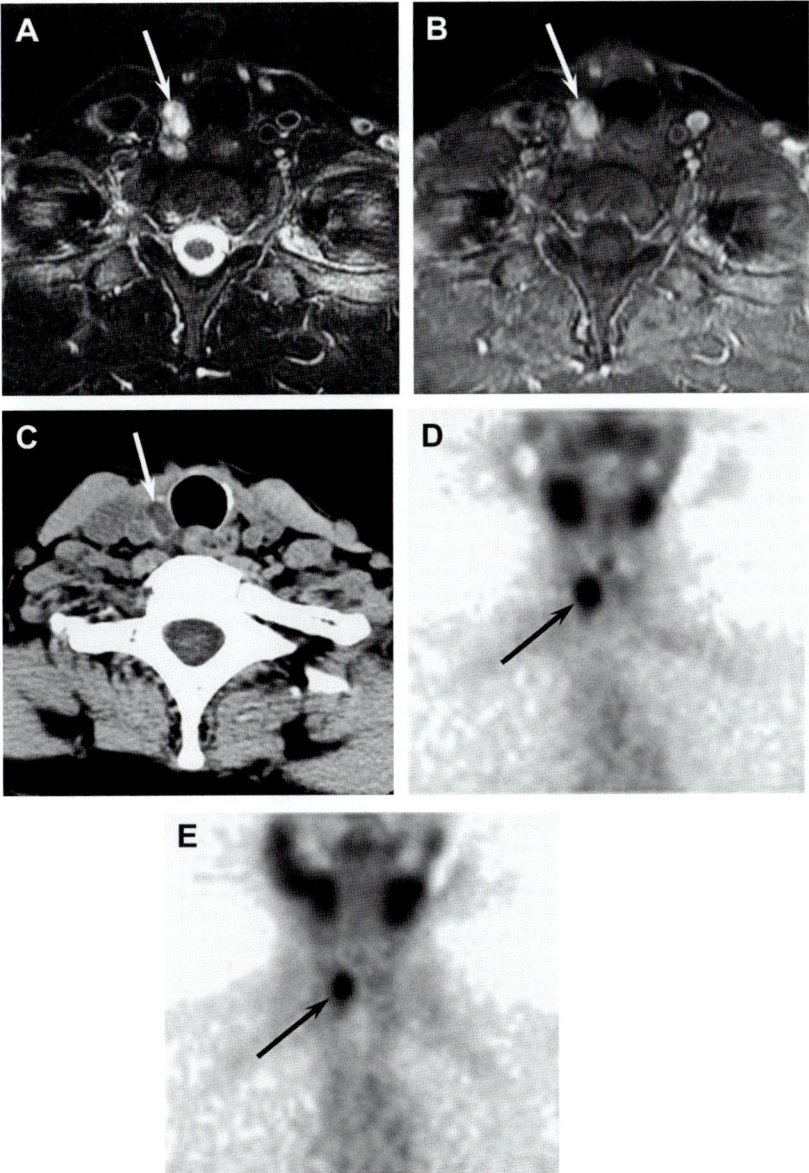

Fig. 9. Parathyroid adenoma. (A) T2-weighted MR image shows a heterogeneous, lobular high-signal mass (*arrow*) in the right tracheoesophageal groove. (B) Corresponding T1-weighted image shows brisk enhancement. (C) Corresponding unenhanced CT image shows the mass to be of low density with scattered calcifications in its rim. Early (D) and late (E) sestamibi images show brisk uptake with retention in the adenoma (*arrows*).

or hyperintense on both T1- and T2-weighted sequences, and must therefore be identified purely on the basis of their abnormal size and location,[33–35] although some authors advocate contrast administration specifically to aide in the detection of these atypical adenomas.[35] On every study, the radiologist should make sure to carefully evaluate the areas above and below the thyroid poles, the carotid artery sheath, the tracheoesophageal groove, and the mediastinum, to make sure that no ectopic parathyroid glands are overlooked.

Parathyroid cysts appear much as cysts elsewhere in the body, demonstrating increased signal on T2-weighted sequences, decreased signal on T1-weighted sequences, and little to no enhancement of a thin wall on postcontrast imaging. The usefulness of MR in diagnosing a parathyroid cyst is in confirming its cystic nature and outlining the anatomy that the cyst traverses.

In cases of parathyroid carcinoma, MR is used as part of a multiple imaging approach to aid in defining the extent of de novo and recurrent disease. MR is optimally suited in helping to navigate the complex anatomy of the neck, delineate the full extent of disease, and aid in planning curative surgery.

Pitfalls

The most significant pitfall in MR imaging of parathyroid disease is concomitant thyroid disease, which has been reported in up to 40% of patients who have hyperparathyroidism.[32] Thyroid glands typically demonstrate increased signal on T2-weighted MR sequences and may mimic the imaging appearance of parathyroid glands. The reverse scenario is equally confusing: intrathyroidal parathyroid glands may have an identical imaging appearance to thyroid nodules.

Knowledge of conventional anatomy, and commonly encountered variant anatomy, is crucial to avoid confusing a normal or aberrant vessel with a parathyroid gland. In certain situation, such as in patients who have markedly aberrant anatomy or abnormal flow dynamics, it has been reported that the addition of gradient echo flow-sensitive pulse sequences may be helpful.[33]

All MR imaging sequences are inherently sensitive to patient motion, including respiratory motion, motion caused by patient swallowing, and normal patient movement, which may give rise to several confusing artifacts, further complicating an already difficult examination. Patients who are likely to move during the examination may be better imaged with CT.

SUMMARY

By far the most common indication for parathyroid imaging is hyperparathyroidism, which is caused by a solitary parathyroid adenoma in the vast majority of patients. The primary function of parathyroid imaging is localization of the abnormal parathyroid gland, enabling the surgeon to pursue a minimally invasive resection. Ultrasound and ^{99m}Tc sestamibi scintigraphy are the mainstays for the preoperative localization of culprit lesions. Multigland disease, caused by double adenoma and parathyroid hyperplasia, is an important cause of operative failure. Because of the technical difficulty, significant morbidity, and cost of reoperation, preoperative parathyroid imaging cannot stop at the identification of an obviously abnormal parathyroid gland, but must carefully examine the entire neck and typical locations of ectopic glands to exclude multigland disease.[31] The emerging modality of SPECT-CT can improve the sensitivity of ^{99m}Tc sestamibi scintigraphy and its use is encouraged when available, particularly in patients who have concurrent thyroid pathology in whom ^{99m}Tc sestamibi imaging results are difficult to accurately interpret.[29]

CT and MR imaging are useful as adjuncts, particularly as anatomic correlates to suspected ectopic glands on ^{99m}Tc sestamibi scintigraphy that are inaccessible to ultrasound. Furthermore, they may be useful in patients who have negative or equivocal ultrasound and ^{99m}Tc sestamibi scintigraphy. 4-D CT may be able to rival the sensitivity of ultrasound and ^{99m}Tc sestamibi scintigraphy, although insufficient data exist to recommend its routine use.[31]

Parathyroid carcinoma is difficult to differentiate from parathyroid adenoma, although a palpable mass, extensive vascular supply, or inseparability from nearby structures should be signs of concern for parathyroid carcinoma. In cases of suspected parathyroid carcinoma, preoperative CT or MR imaging is recommended for surgical planning.

REFERENCES

1. Johnson NA, Tublin ME, Ogilvie JB. Parathyroid imaging: technique and role in the preoperative evaluation of primary hyperparathyroidism. AJR Am J Roentgenol 2007;188(6):1706–15.
2. Mettler FA, Guiberteau MJ. Essentials of nuclear medicine imaging. 5th edition. Philadelphia: Saunders/Elsevier; 2006.
3. Nguyen BD. Parathyroid imaging with Tc-99m sestamibi planar and SPECT scintigraphy. Radiographics 1999;19(3):601–14 [discussion: 615–06].
4. Smith JR, Oates ME. Radionuclide imaging of the parathyroid glands: patterns, pearls, and pitfalls. Radiographics 2004;24(4):1101–15.
5. Akerstrom G, Malmaeus J, Bergstrom R. Surgical anatomy of human parathyroid glands. Surgery 1984;95(1):14–21.
6. Meilstrup JW. Ultrasound examination of the parathyroid glands. Otolaryngol Clin North Am 2004;37(4):763–78, ix.
7. Perez-Monte JE, Brown ML, Shah AN, et al. Parathyroid adenomas: accurate detection and localization with Tc-99m sestamibi SPECT. Radiology 1996;201(1):85–91.
8. Uruno T, Kebebew E. How to localize parathyroid tumors in primary hyperparathyroidism? J Endocrinol Invest 2006;29(9):840–7.
9. van Dalen A, Smit CP, van Vroonhoven TJ, et al. Minimally invasive surgery for solitary parathyroid adenomas in patients with primary hyperparathyroidism: role of US with supplemental CT. Radiology 2001;220(3):631–9.

10. Braunwald E. Harrison's principles of internal medicine. 15th edition. New York: McGraw-Hill; 2001.
11. Romero-Urquhart G, Mishkin FS, Vasinrapee P. Parathyroid adenoma. Available at: http://www.emedicine.com/radio/topic525.htm. Accessed May 1, 2007.
12. Fitzpatrick LA. Hypercalcemia in the multiple endocrine neoplasia syndromes. Endocrinol Metab Clin North Am 1989;18(3):741–52.
13. Herfarth KK, Wells SA Jr. Parathyroid glands and the multiple endocrine neoplasia syndromes and familial hypocalciuric hypercalcemia. Semin Surg Oncol 1997;13(2):114–24.
14. Mallette LE. Management of hyperparathyroidism in the multiple endocrine neoplasia syndromes and other familial endocrinopathies. Endocrinol Metab Clin North Am 1994;23(1):19–36.
15. Skogseid B, Rastad J, Oberg K. Multiple endocrine neoplasia type 1. Clinical features and screening. Endocrinol Metab Clin North Am 1994;23(1):1–18.
16. Barraclough BM, Barraclough BH. Ultrasound of the thyroid and parathyroid glands. World J Surg 2000;24(2):158–65.
17. Carpenter JM, Michaelson PG, Lidner TK, et al. Parathyromatosis. Ear Nose Throat J 2007;86(1):21.
18. Kollmorgen CF, Aust MR, Ferreiro JA, et al. Parathyromatosis: a rare yet important cause of persistent or recurrent hyperparathyroidism. Surgery 1994;116(1):111–5.
19. Kendrick ML, Charboneau JW, Curlee KJ, et al. Risk of parathyromatosis after fine-needle aspiration. Am Surg 2001;67(3):290–3 [discussion: 293–4].
20. Beyer TD, Solorzano CC, Starr F, et al. Parathyroidectomy outcomes according to operative approach. Am J Surg 2007;193(3):368–72 [discussion: 372–63].
21. Howe JR. Minimally invasive parathyroid surgery. Surg Clin North Am 2000;80(5):1399–426.
22. Kamaya A, Quon A, Jeffrey RB. Sonography of the abnormal parathyroid gland. Ultrasound Q 2006;22(4):253–62.
23. Ryan JA Jr, Lee FT. Maximizing outcomes while minimizing exploration in hyperparathyroidism using localization tests. Arch Surg 2004;139(8):838–42 [discussion: 842–33].
24. Smit PC, Borel Rinkes IH, van Dalen A, et al. Direct, minimally invasive adenomectomy for primary hyperparathyroidism: an alternative to conventional neck exploration? Ann Surg 2000;231(4):559–65.
25. Mackie GC, Schlicht SM. Accurate localization of supernumerary mediastinal parathyroid adenomas by a combination of structural and functional imaging. Australas Radiol 2004;48(3):392–7.
26. De Feo ML, Colagrande S, Biagini C, et al. Parathyroid glands: combination of (99m)Tc MIBI scintigraphy and US for demonstration of parathyroid glands and nodules. Radiology 2000;214(2):393–402.
27. Ruda JM, Hollenbeak CS, Stack BC Jr. A systematic review of the diagnosis and treatment of primary hyperparathyroidism from 1995 to 2003. Otolaryngol Head Neck Surg 2005;132(3):359–72.
28. Coakley AJ, Kettle AG, Wells CP, et al. 99Tcm sestamibi—a new agent for parathyroid imaging. Nucl Med Commun 1989;10(11):791–4.
29. Lavely WC, Goetze S, Friedman KP, et al. Comparison of SPECT/CT, SPECT, and planar imaging with single- and dual-phase (99m)Tc-sestamibi parathyroid scintigraphy. J Nucl Med 2007;48(7):1084–9.
30. Vattimo A, Bertelli P, Cintorino M, et al. Identification of Hürthle cell tumor by single-injection, double-phase scintigraphy with technetium-99m-sestamibi. J Nucl Med 1995;36(5):778–82.
31. Rodgers SE, Hunter GJ, Hamberg LM, et al. Improved preoperative planning for directed parathyroidectomy with 4-dimensional computed tomography. Surgery 2006;140(6):932–40 [discussion: 940–31].
32. Clark P, Wooldridge T, Kleinpeter K, et al. Providing optimal preoperative localization for recurrent parathyroid carcinoma: a combined parathyroid scintigraphy and computed tomography approach. Clin Nucl Med 2004;29(11):681–4.
33. Lee VS, Spritzer CE. MR imaging of abnormal parathyroid glands. AJR Am J Roentgenol 1998;170(4):1097–103.
34. Lee VS, Spritzer CE, Coleman RE, et al. The complementary roles of fast spin-echo MR imaging and double-phase 99m Tc-sestamibi scintigraphy for localization of hyperfunctioning parathyroid glands. AJR Am J Roentgenol 1996;167(6):1555–62.
35. Lopez Hanninen E, Vogl TJ, Steinmuller T, et al. Preoperative contrast-enhanced MRI of the parathyroid glands in hyperparathyroidism. Invest Radiol 2000;35(7):426–30.

Parathyroid Surgery: What the Radiologists Need to Know

Richard O. Wein, MD, FACS[a,*], Randal S. Weber, MD, FACS[b]

KEYWORDS

- Hyperparathyroidism • Parathyroid adenoma
- Parathyroid hyperplasia • Parathyroidectomy
- Intraoperative PTH • MIP

Hyperparathyroidism represents by a varied spectrum of presentations, from those individuals who have overt symptoms directly attributable to hypercalcemia to those who are asymptomatic at diagnosis. Indications for surgical intervention in the asymptomatic population have changed as the long-term experience with these patients has grown. Over the last 10 years, surgery for primary hyperparathyroidism, in the setting of a single localized adenoma, has evolved for some surgeons from a standard four-gland exploration into a radioguided, minimally invasive outpatient procedure. Additionally, technological developments, such as the rapid intraoperative assessment of parathyroid hormone (PTH) levels, can be used to guide the effectiveness of a surgical procedure while the patient remains under anesthesia. Medications such as calcimimetics, agents that reduce the PTH secretion, may have a role in the treatment of selected cases of hyperparathyroidism. Despite the progress made in the technology associated with the surgical management of this diagnosis, however, patients requiring reoperation for persistent hypercalcemia continue to remain a challenge for even the most experienced surgeons. Use of additional imaging techniques to aid localization and a detailed understanding of the anatomy can be critical to a successful operative outcome. This article discusses the pertinent issues that surround the current surgical management of parathyroid disease with a focus on epidemiology, surgical anatomy, and operative strategies.

EPIDEMIOLOGY

PTH acts to increase serum calcium levels by working at the level of the bone, kidney, and gastrointestinal tract. Hyperparathyroidism reflects the adjustment of the body's set point for serum calcium at a level above normal. The calcium-sensing receptor (CaR) of the parathyroid gland is the principal regulator of PTH secretion. Activation of this receptor, with changes in serum calcium levels, also affects calcitonin secretion and urinary calcium secretion.[1]

Hyperparathyroidism presents in three forms: primary, secondary, and tertiary. Primary hyperparathyroidism is characterized by hypercalcemia in the setting of an elevated PTH level. The estimated prevalence of primary hyperparathyroidism in North America is 1 in 1000 patients and the highest incidence is in postmenopausal women.[2] Secondary hyperparathyroidism is seen in association with longstanding renal failure and treatment focuses on medical management with a subset of patients ultimately requiring surgery. Tertiary hyperparathyroidism occurs in the setting of secondary hyperparathyroidism when the parathyroid glands lose the ability for feedback regulation.

---

[a] Department of Otolaryngology–Head and Neck Surgery, Tufts Medical Center, 750 Washington Street, Box #850, Boston, MA 02111, USA
[b] Department of Head and Neck Surgery, Unit 441, University of Texas M.D. Anderson Cancer Center, 1515 Holcombe Boulevard, Houston, TX 77030, USA
* Corresponding author.
E-mail address: rwein@tufts-nemc.org (R.O. Wein).

Primary hyperparathyroidism is more common in females (3:1 ratio) and represents a single adenoma in greater than four fifths of all cases. Most patients are asymptomatic at presentation and are ultimately diagnosed when a serum calcium level is assessed for other reasons. The typical age of presentation is during the fifth and sixth decades of life. A history of long-term lithium use may be associated with the development of primary hyperparathyroidism.

EMBRYOLOGY AND BASICS

The parathyroid glands are derived from the third (inferior glands associated with the thymus) and fourth (superior glands) branchial pouches; this is pertinent to surgical management of the glands and the assessment for missing parathyroid adenomas.

The typical parathyroid gland weighs between 30 and 65 mg and is oval with a mahogany-tan color. It is composed of chief (producing PTH), intermediate, and oxyphilic cells. The vast majority of parathyroid adenomas are the result of expansion of the chief cell population; however, a limited percentage of adenomas represent oncocytic and lipoadenomatous variants. Four glands are normally present in 84% of patients. Three percent of patients are reported to have only three glands and as many as 13% of patients have been noted to have more than four glands.[3,4]

The typical location of the superior parathyroid glands is 1 cm superior to the junction of the recurrent laryngeal nerve (RLN) and inferior thyroid artery. The inferior glands, which are more variable in anatomic localization, approximate the inferolateral or posterior thyroid pole in 50% of cases and are within the thyrothymic fat in 24% of cases.[3]

In a review of more than 20,000 cases of hyperparathyroidism from 1995 to 2003 performed by Ruda and colleagues[5] the reported frequency of specific pathologies was the following: solitary adenoma, 88.90%; double adenoma, 4.14%; multiple gland hyperplasia disease, 5.74%; parathyroid carcinoma, 0.74%.

Ectopic locations where aberrant parathyroid glands can be located include: para/retroesophageal region, intrathyroidal (more commonly superior), carotid sheath (more commonly inferior), associated with the thymus, and mediastinal.

Patients who have parathyroid carcinoma calcium tend to present with calcium levels greater than 14 mg/dL with 80% of patients being symptomatic from the hypercalcemia at diagnosis. Based on the 22-year review at M.D. Anderson Cancer Center, there was noted to be a slight male predominance with the mean age of presentation 47 years. Most patients initially presented with locally invasive disease without distant metastasis. Locoregional recurrence was common and all deaths were considered related to hypercalcemia.[6]

Assessment for variants of the multiple endocrine neoplasia (MEN) syndromes may require evaluation in the hypercalcemic population. These variants include MEN1 (parathyroid hyperplasia, pituitary adenoma, and pancreatic cell tumors), MEN2A (parathyroid hyperplasia, MTC, pheochromocytoma), non-MEN familial hyperparathyroidism, and benign familial hypocalciuric hypercalcemia (BFHH). In BFHH, a defect in PTH sensing in renal tubules within the kidney results in hypercalcemia.

INDICATIONS FOR SURGERY

Symptomatic patients are offered surgery with the goal of stabilizing or resolving the issues that lead to their initial presentation. Most hyperparathyroid patients are diagnosed when they are asymptomatic. As such, the indications for the surgical management of these patients were established. In 1990, the National Institutes of Health (NIH) Consensus Conference on Asymptomatic Primary Hyperparathyroidism established guidelines indicating parameters for parathyroidectomy (**Box 1**).[7]

In 2002 the NIH Workshop on Primary Hyperparathyroidism re-examined the prior guidelines and changed many of the original recommendations.[8] The criterion for total serum calcium concentration was decreased to 1 mg/dL (from 1.6 mg/dL) above the upper limits of normal. Bone density at the lumbar spine, hip, or distal radius greater than 2.5 standard deviations below peak bone mass was also established as an indication for parathyroidectomy. The original recommendations of intervening for 24-hour urinary calcium greater than 400 mg, for the reduction of creatinine clearance by 30% (compared with age-matched subjects), when medical surveillance is not desirable or possible, and for age less than 50 years remained unchanged. Approximately 50% of asymptomatic patients fulfill one of the previously described indications for surgery. Patients who do not have an indication for surgery, or who desire not to pursue surgical intervention, should be followed long term to assess for the development of a surgical indication or symptoms related to their diagnosis.

The role that calcimimetics will have on future indications for surgery in the asymptomatic patients is yet to be determined.[9]

HISTORY AND PHYSICAL EXAMINATION

In the symptomatic patient, the duration and intensity of the patient's presenting symptoms should

> **Box 1**
> **Indications for parathyroidectomy**
>
> The 1990 Guidelines specifying indications for parathyroidectomy in the asymptomatic patient and the 2002 modifications to the original guidelines.
>
> Serum calcium >12 mg/dL (or ≥1.6 mg/dL greater than the referenced upper limit of normal)
>
> - 2002 modification: serum calcium decreased from 1.6 mg/dL to 1.0 mg/dL above the upper limit of normal
>
> Marked hypercalciuria (24-hour urinary calcium >400 mg/d)
>
> Overt manifestations (such as nephrolithiasis, osteitis fibrosa cystica, or classic neuromuscular disease)
>
> Markedly reduced cortical bone density (z-score < −2)
>
> - 2002 modification: bone density at the lumbar spine, hip, or distal radius greater than 2.5 standard deviations below peak mass (using t-scoring instead of z-score)
>
> Reduced creatinine clearance (by greater than 30% compared with age-matched cohorts) in the absence of any other cause
>
> Age <50 years
>
> Patients in whom surveillance with close clinical follow-up is not possible or desired
>
> *Data from* NIH Conference. Diagnosis and management of asymptomatic primary hyperparathyroidism: consensus development conference statement. Ann Intern Med 1991;114:593–7; and Bilezikian JP, Potts Jr JT, Fuleihan Gel-H, et al. Summary statement from a workshop on asymptomatic primary hyperparathyroidism: a perspective for the 21st century. J Clin Endocrinol Metab 2002;87(12):535–61.

be reviewed. Diagnoses, such as hypertension and peptic ulcer disease, that may or may not be related to the diagnosis of hyperparathyroidism, may be noted within the patient's history. Symptoms of fatigue, depression, memory problems, abdominal pain, constipation, and pain in other parts of the body can be associated with hypercalcemia. A history of prior low-dose irradiation is associated with an increased risk for developing hyperparathyroidism. Nephrolithiasis is the most common presentation of symptomatic disease and is noted in approximately one fifth of patients who have primary hyperparathyroidism. History of prior thiazide diuretic or lithium and prior consumption of calcium and vitamins A and D should also be assessed.

Issues of importance when assessing a patient for parathyroid surgery include a history of prior neck or thyroid-based surgery and the patient's ability to extend the neck. The presence of coexisting thyroid pathology (nodule, goiter) could make a procedure more technically challenging and may require preoperative ultrasound assessment and fine needle aspiration. True vocal cord function and assessment of the airway allows the surgeon to appreciate the patient's baseline vocal cord function in particular in the setting of revision parathyroid surgery. Overall the results of physical examination, as it relates to the diagnosis of hyperparathyroidism, are typically unremarkable.

PREOPERATIVE EVALUATION

After establishing the diagnosis of hyperparathyroidism with the identification of elevated intact PTH and serum calcium levels, additional preoperative labs should be considered. Checking creatinine and BUN levels allows for assessment of baseline renal function. Additional labs that should be considered include albumin, magnesium, chloride (typically high), and phosphorus (typically low). An elevated alkaline phosphatase may indicate a risk for postoperative bone hunger requiring the need for aggressive postoperative supplementation and close monitoring. Assessment of a 24-hour urine sample for calcium allows for evaluation of the potential diagnosis of BFHH, for which surgery is not indicated. Hypercalcemia of malignancy should be excluded as part of the work-up and is typically not associated with elevated level of PTH.

Preoperative tests to aid in the localization are numerous and include ultrasonography, CT, MR imaging, and technetium-99m (^{99m}Tc) sestamibi. The goal of localization is to first identify if the cause is a discrete single adenoma to aid in operative planning. Given the potential anatomic variability of the parathyroid glands, use of an imaging modality with excellent sensitivity for localization can significantly increase the success of the proposed procedure, reduce operative time, reduce complication rates, and enable the consideration for use of minimally invasive surgical techniques.

The current initial imaging of choice for the detection of parathyroid adenomas is ^{99m}Tc sestamibi scanning (**Fig. 1**). The reported sensitivity for double-phase ^{99m}Tc sestamibi scanning is greater than 85% for the detection of parathyroid adenomas, whereas the sensitivity for hyperplasia is around 50%. The accuracy of scanning is directly

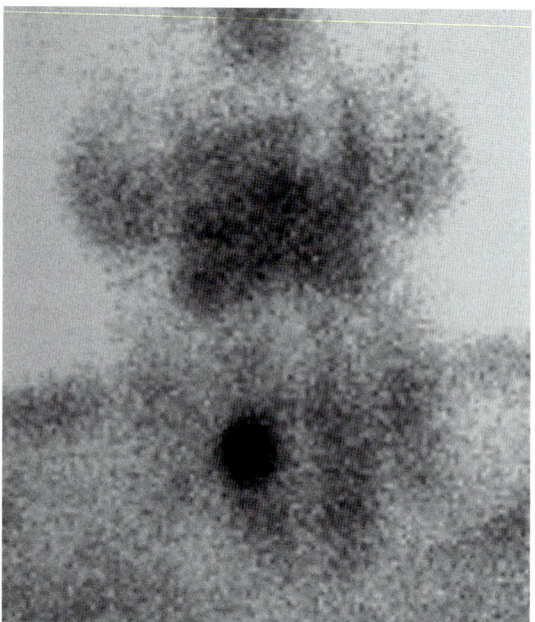

Fig. 1. Typical appearance of a sestamibi scan localizing a parathyroid adenoma that approximates the right upper pole of the thyroid.

related to the size of the adenoma being studied. Thyroid pathology, such as goiters, adenomas, or carcinomas, may impact on the accuracy of the assessment. ^{99}Tc-labeled sestamibi scanning can be combined with single photon emission computed tomography imaging resulting in the generation of a three-dimensional image that may assist with spatial orientation when attempting to localize an adenoma. Reported sensitivity is as high as 88.9% for patients who have a solitary adenoma, yet sensitivity decreases to 45% with multigland disease.[5] The study misses approximately 87% of patients who have multigland disease, however.[10] Success with the technique is dictated by oxyphil cell population of a specific adenoma.[11] The sensitivity of the assay is less successful in scenarios of revision surgery, for lesions within the mediastinum, and in patients who are morbidly obese.[12]

The advantage of ultrasound is that it is noninvasive and easily tolerated. It has a reported sensitivity of 79% in patients who have solitary adenomas in the setting of primary hyperparathyroidism yet decreases to 35% with multigland disease.[5] Sensitivity is limited when assessing for ectopic parathyroid within the mediastinum or tracheoesophageal groove; however, with larger adenomas (>1 g) sensitivity can approach 95%. Intraoperative ultrasound is advocated by some authors[13] and considered particularly helpful in use with young adults.[14] Ultrasound also has the capacity for synchronous preoperative evaluation of thyroid pathology that may require treatment at the time of parathyroid surgery.

CT scanning with contrast can be performed with thin cuts and has the capacity to assess the mediastinum; however, sensitivity is limited for parathyroid adenomas or hyperplasia.

MR imaging with contrast has superior soft tissue imaging capabilities when compared with CT and may be particularly helpful in identifying ectopic parathyroid glands. Sensitivity is reported to be greater than 75% for localization adenomas. MR imaging combined with the use of selective venous sampling has been advocated in the setting of the reoperative parathyroidectomy as complimentary imaging modalities with good accuracy at predicting the site of recurrent or persistent focus when both are positive.[15]

In previously operated patients, imaging requirements may necessitate obtaining multiple studies using the attributes of many of the modalities already discussed. Positron emission tomography scanning may have a role in these scenarios also.

OPERATIVE ANATOMY

The parathyroid gland is identified as a flattened oval, a light brown to tan colored structured that is distinct from the surrounding soft tissues of the neck when examining a hemostatic operative field (**Fig. 2**). Differentiation from lymph nodes and components of the thyroid gland can be challenging. The parathyroid glands, upper and lower, are closely associated to the RLN (**Fig. 3**). The upper glands are dorsal to a coronal plane created by the path of the RLN, whereas the lower glands are ventral to this plane.[12] The lower gland is typically located within 1 cm of the inferolateral aspect of the lower pole of the ipsilateral thyroid lobe. The upper gland is typically located at the cricothyroid region approximately 1 cm superior to the junction of the RLN and inferior thyroid artery posterolateral to the upper pole of the ipsilateral thyroid lobe.

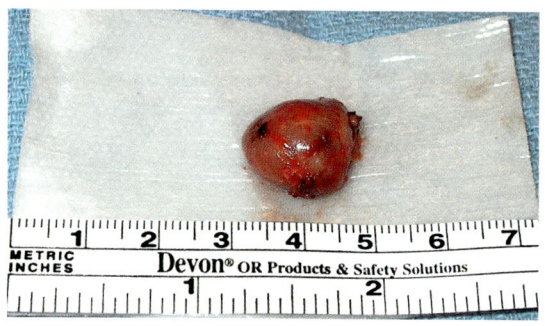

Fig. 2. Parathyroid adenoma after removal.

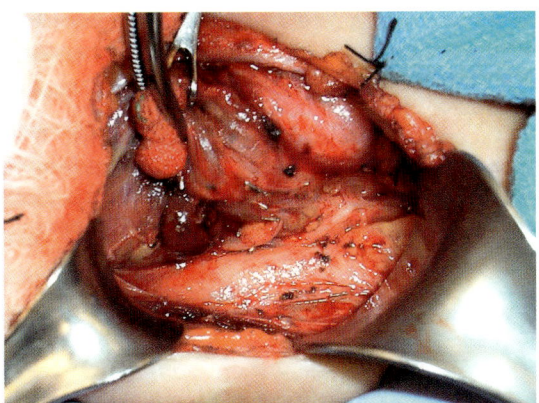

Fig. 3. The operative approach to the right neck in the setting of persistent hypercalcemia after prior surgical intervention. The thyroid gland is retracted to the midline. The recurrent laryngeal nerve enters the operative field inferiorly and tracks superiorly in the tracheoesophageal groove. The carotid sheath contents are lateral to the nerve and at the superior pole of the right thyroid lobe (at 8 o'clock) is a mahogany lobular mass representing the parathyroid adenoma.

Ectopic locations associated with the upper and lower glands tend to follow paths consistent with the embryologic descent. Upper glands tend to be located posteriorly, such as in the retropharyngeal and retroesophageal spaces, and extend into the posterior mediastinum, whereas lower glands may be found more anteriorly in locations such as thymus and anterior mediastinum. The anatomic location of the inferior parathyroid gland tends to be more variable secondary to the longer path of descent required for these glands. Intrathyroidal presentations of parathyroid tissue are estimated to occur in only 1% of cases and occur more commonly with lower glands. The predominant blood supply to the parathyroid glands is the inferior thyroid artery. The superior parathyroid glands also receive a portion of their blood supply from anastomotic branches of the superior parathyroid artery.

OPERATIVE CONSIDERATIONS

At the time of surgery, maintaining hemostasis is critical to parathyroidectomy. Use of loupe magnification can assist with the surgeon with visualizing subtle anatomic structures. Nerve integrity monitoring, in particular during reoperative scenarios, can assist in identification and preservation of the recurrent laryngeal nerve.

For single gland disease, removal of the intact adenoma is the goal of surgery. Surgical strategies for the management of parathyroid hyperplasia include four-gland exploration with resection of three and one half versus four glands. In four-gland resections, reimplantation may be performed in the neck or arm. In addition, cryopreservation is possible with capacity for future reimplantation. The aggressiveness of the surgical approach in hyperplasia can be tailored to the virulence of the underlying pathology. Presentations such as MEN1, familial hyperparathyroidism, and secondary hyperparathyroidism are considered more virulent in course and require a more aggressive surgical approach, such as four-gland resection with removal of thymus, central neck dissection, and reimplantation. Less virulent forms of hyperplasia, such as double adenoma, spontaneous (nonsyndromic) four-gland hyperplasia, and MEN2A, may require only range removal of enlarged glands to three and one half gland resection.[12]

The standard approach to parathyroidectomy, until the advent of minimally invasive and radio-guided protocols, included bilateral neck exploration with four-gland identification. Patients who have negative sestamibi scans are typically excluded from minimally invasive parathyroidectomy-based protocols. Modifications on the technique included unilateral neck exploration in specific settings. Postoperative normocalcemia has been reported to be 95% in patients undergoing this approach.[5]

The management of operable parathyroid carcinoma includes en bloc resection, hemithyroidectomy with central neck dissection, and postoperative radiation therapy in an attempt to achieve local control of disease.[6]

OPERATIVE ASSISTANCE TECHNIQUES

Intraoperative intact PTH is performed as sequential assay of intact PTH levels that are compared with pre-incisional or pre-removal levels. After removal of the adenoma is accomplished, levels may be drawn at 5-, 10-, or 20-minute post-removal intervals. If subsequent intact PTH levels are reduced by greater than 50%, the procedure is generally considered successful and closure of the operative site is performed. The technique has also been described as an aid in cases requiring removal of multiple parathyroid glands or in the reoperative patient. The technique was found to be useful in 60% of cases requiring conversion to bilateral neck exploration achieving postoperative normocalcemia of 98% in those cases with a true-positive rate of 98%.[5] The technique is not uniformly used and there are advocates suggesting use with every case[10] just as there are critics of the technique.[16] Assay at 10 minutes can result in a false-positive interpretation (with bilateral neck exploration pursued) that would have resolved to a greater than 50% reduction of preoperative levels at 20 minutes in situations in which patients are slow metabolizers, are renal insufficient, or had large adenomas of 3 g or greater.[5] In the setting of negative (8%) or incorrect (12%) sestamibi scanning, in one study intraoperative intact PTH changed operative management in 82% (86/105) of patients by demonstrating incomplete resection (in patients with incorrect single-focus sestamibi scanning results) or multiglandular disease, and allowed avoidance of unnecessary bilateral neck exploration.[10]

Minimally invasive radio-guided parathyroidectomy is another approach to parathyroidectomy. A preoperative dose of sestamibi is given to the patient that allows for intraoperative use of gamma probe to aid localization. Postoperative normocalcemia has been reported to be achieved in 97% of cases when using this technique.[5] As with all techniques, there are critics of this approach,[16] and it is typically used when a single adenoma is identified preoperatively. Parathyroidectomy with minimally invasive protocols can be performed with local anesthesia, whereas standard multi-gland exploration typically requires general anesthesia.

Minimally invasive parathyroidectomy (MIP) is performed through a 2-cm lateral focused mini-incision. It is performed for primary hyperparathyroidism when a preoperative sestamibi localizes an adenoma. A preoperative ultrasound is also performed to aid incision placement. Approximately 50% of patients are capable of undergoing MIP with surgeons experienced in the technique.[17] Intraoperative PTH may be used with MIP; however, some authors argue it is not necessary in the setting of good preoperative localization studies.[18] In a study examining MIP (incision length <2.5 cm) with intraoperative PTH a 9% rate of unnecessary conversion to bilateral neck exploration was reported based on 10-minute sample readings of PTH.[18]

Endoscopic parathyroidectomy has been reported an also has its critics.[16] An additional strategy used to aid intraoperative localization is the use of an intravenous infusion of methylene blue. Abnormal parathyroid glands stain dark to light blue and can assist the surgeon in cases such as those with ectopic glands.[19]

Frozen section is a topic of controversy when performing parathyroidectomy. In one study gross examination by experienced parathyroid surgeons demonstrated the correct identification of parathyroid in 94% of cases when specimens were subject to frozen section confirmatory evaluation. The authors concluded that frozen section was unnecessary in routine situations.[20] Frozen section differentiation between parathyroid hyperplasia versus adenoma remains a challenge. The expense of frozen section assessment is greater than 10 times the cost of a rapid intraoperative PTH assay at some institutions. Some advocate use of frozen sections for the infrequent thyroid surgeon, multiple gland disease, ectopic glands, reoperated neck, and with technically difficult surgeries.[20]

REOPERATIVE SETTING

Hyperparathyroidism after prior attempt at parathyroidectomy is a challenging issue to address. When the problem is related to a missed adenoma, the locations where reoperation is most likely to detect the missing adenoma are the thyrothymic horn, lower thymus, paraesophageal/retroesophageal region, associated with the carotid sheath, or at previously described normal anatomic locations specific to the gland. As mentioned, intrathyroidal presentation is uncommon and rates of incidence vary within the literature. Use of thyroid lobectomy in the setting of missing adenoma is controversial.

Recurrent laryngeal nerve monitoring and intraoperative PTH have been advocated in reoperative scenarios because the success of treatment decreases with each reoperation. Surgical management in this situation requires establishing the standard landmarks for superior and inferior glands, resectioning thymic fat from anterior mediastinum, following the recurrent laryngeal nerves and dissecting out paratracheal tissue bilaterally, opening both carotid sheaths from hyoid to mediastinum, dissecting in the retropharyngeal plane, and possible thyroidectomy.

POSTOPERATIVE CONSIDERATIONS

Complications of parathyroidectomy invariably include hypocalcemia. Hungry bone syndrome characterized by hypophosphatemia and hypocalcemia in patients who have longstanding hyperparathyroidism with extensive bony resorption may require extensive calcium supplementation. Recurrent laryngeal nerve weakness or paralysis manifests in changes in vocal quality and may also be associated with dysphagia and aspiration.

Calcium supplementation, either intravenous or oral, may be required. Cardiac monitoring should be considered in patients actively requiring supplementation because of the risk for arrhythmia. Vitamin D and magnesium supplementation may also be required in the postoperative setting of severe hypocalcemia.

Although the trend has been toward outpatient surgery for the management of uncomplicated adenoma removal with minimally invasive techniques, more extensive procedures may still warrant inpatient postoperative management. Opinions on this topic vary as widely as the varying surgical approaches.[21]

The choice of postoperative calcium and PTH assessment with selective treatment of hypocalcemia versus empiric treatment is also an area of debate. Some advocates state that patients undergoing subtotal parathyroidectomy for hyperplasia should have an 8-hour postoperative PTH level greater than or equal to 15 pg/mL to be considered at low risk for developing postoperative hypocalcemia. Patients who have PTH levels less than 15 pg/mL (1.6 pmol/L) are considered at higher risk for developing hypocalcemia (75%) and should have empiric treatment initiated with calcium and calcitriol.[22]

COMPLICATED PATIENTS WHO HAVE PERSISTENT HYPERCALCEMIA

Calcimimetics act to amplify the sensitivity of the CaR, which is the primary regulator of PTH secretion, to changes in extracellular calcium levels. The impact of these medications in patients who have recurrent postoperative hypercalcemia is yet to be clarified. Success has been noted with the use of calcimimetics in patients who have secondary hyperparathyroidism in the reduction of PTH, calcium, and phosphorus levels, in addition to a reduced risk for fracture and hospitalization secondary to cardiovascular complications.[1]

Selective alcohol embolization of parathyroid tissue has been described yet remains controversial. Ultrasound-guided needle ablation in patients considered at high risk for surgical intervention has also been described. Some authors have advocated that MR imaging and selective venous sampling are complementary techniques in reoperative patients and have been reported to assist in successful outcomes in 93% of patients.[9] Selective venous sampling has a reported sensitivity of 90% in scenarios of recurrent or persistent hyperparathyroidism requiring reoperation.[23]

Patients who have parathyroid carcinoma may be considered candidates for postoperative radiation therapy. Medical management with bisphosphonates, calcitonin, and calcimimetics may have a role in addressing persistent postoperative hypercalcemia. Overall 5- and 10-year survival is 85% and 49%, respectively.[24]

SUMMARY

There are various techniques to assist in the localization of abnormal parathyroid tissue; however, surgeon experience remains among the most important factors to achieve the desired results from surgical intervention. Several operative approaches and use of various intraoperative techniques to assist the surgeon have been developed over the last decade and there is controversy within the literature about the necessity and expense associated with the use of these techniques.

REFERENCES

1. Torres PU. Cinacalcet HCl: a novel treatment for secondary hyperparathyroidism caused by chronic kidney disease. J Ren Nutr 2006;16:253–8.
2. Boonstra CE, Jackson CE. Serum calcium survey for hyperparathyroidism: results in 50,000 clinic patients. Am J Clin Pathol 1971;55:523–6.
3. Akerstrom G, Malmaeus J, Bergstrom R. Surgical anatomy of human parathyroid glands. Surgery 1984;95:14–21.
4. Pattou FN, Pellissier LC, Noel C, et al. Supernumerary parathyroid glands: frequency and surgical significance in treatment of renal hyperparathyroidism. World J Surg 2000;24:1330–4.
5. Ruda JM, Hollenbeak CS, Stack BC Jr. A systematic review of the diagnosis and treatment of primary hyperparathyroidism from 1995 to 2003. Otolaryngol Head Neck Surg 2005;132:359–72.
6. Busaidy NL, Jimenez C, Habra MA, et al. Parathyroid carcinoma: a 22-year experience. Head Neck 2004;26:716–26.
7. NIH Conference. Diagnosis and management of asymptomatic primary hyperparathyroidism: consensus development conference statement. Ann Intern Med 1991;114:593–7.
8. Bilezikian JP, Potts JT Jr, Fuleihan Gel-H, et al. Summary statement from a workshop on asymptomatic primary hyperparathyroidism: a perspective for the 21st century. J Clin Endocrinol Metab 2002;87(12):535–61.
9. Elder GJ. Parathyroidectomy in the calcimimetic era. Nephrology (Carlton) 2005;10(5):511–5.
10. Carneiro-Pla DM, Solorzano CC, Irvin GL. Consequences of targeted parathyroidectomy guided by localization studies without intraoperative parathyroid hormone monitoring. J Am Coll Surg 2006;202:715–22.
11. Bleier BS, LiVolsi VA, Chalian AA, et al. Technetium Tc 99m sestamibi sensitivity in oxyphil cell-dominant parathyroid adenomas. Arch Otolaryngol Head Neck Surg 2006;132:779–82.
12. Randolph GW, Urken ML. Surgical management of primary hyperparathyroidism. In: Randolph GW, editor. Surgery of the thyroid and the parathyroid glands. Philadelphia: Elsevier Science; 2003. p. 507–28.

13. Solorzano CC, Carneiro-Pla DM, Irvin GL III. Surgeon-performed ultrasonography as the initial and only localizing study in sporadic primary hyperparathyroidism. J Am Coll Surg 2006;202:18–24.
14. Joshua B, Feinmesser R, Ulanovski D, et al. Primary hyperparathyroidism in young adults. Otolaryngol Head Neck Surg 2004;131:628–32.
15. Rotstein L, Irish J, Gullane P, et al. Reoperative parathyroidectomy in the era of localization technology. Head Neck 1998;20:535–9.
16. Ferzli G, Patel S, Graham A, et al. Three new tools for parathyroid surgery: expensive and unnecessary? J Am Coll Surg 2004;198:349–51.
17. Soon PSH, Yeh MW, Sywak MS, et al. Minimally invasive parathyroidectomy using the lateral focused mini-incision approach: is there a learning curve for surgeons experienced in the open procedure? J Am Coll Surg 2007;204:91–5.
18. Stalberg P, Sidhu S, Sywak M, et al. Intraoperative parathyroid hormone measurement during minimally invasive parathyroidectomy: does it "value-add" to decision making? J Am Coll Surg 2006;203:1–6.
19. Kuriloff DB, Sanborn KV. Rapid intraoperative localization of parathyroid glands utilizing methylene blue infusion. Otolaryngol Head Neck Surg 2004; 131:616–22.
20. Dewan AK, Kapadia SB, Hollenbeak CS, et al. Is routine frozen section necessary for parathyroid surgery? Otolaryngol Head Neck Surg 2005;133:857–62.
21. Norman J, Aronson K. Outpatient surgery and the differences seen in the morbidly obese. Otolaryngol Head Neck Surg 2007;136:282–6.
22. Chia SA, Weisman RA, Tieu D, et al. Prospective study of perioperative factors predicting hypocalcemia after thyroid and parathyroid surgery. Arch Otolaryngol Head Neck Surg 2006;132:41–5.
23. Seehofer D, Steinmuller T, Rayes N, et al. Parathyroid hormone venous sampling before reoperative surgery in renal hyperparathyroidism: comparison of noninvasive localization procedures and review of the literature. Arch Surg 2004;139(12):1331–8.
24. Lumachi F, Basso SM, Basso U. Parathyroid cancer: etiology, clinical presentation, and treatment. Anticancer Res 2006;26:4803–7.

Index

Note: Page numbers of article titles are in **boldface** type.

A

Adenoma, parathyroid, 537, 538, 542, 547, 554
    ectopic, 544
Anaplastic thyroid carcinoma, 454, 470–471
    clinical presentation of, 497
    pathology of, 497

C

Calcimimetics, in hyperparathyroidism, 557
Cervical lymph node(s), anatomy of, 479, 480
    calcification of, 483
    classification of, 479
    hyperechoic, 482, 483
    hyperplastic, 481
    in thyroid cancer, sonographic imaging of, **479–489**
    metastatic, 481–483, 484
    normal, 480–481
Colon cancer, metastatic, papillary thyroid carcinoma in, 513, 514
Cornea, in Graves disease, 530
Cross-sectional imaging, of thyroid gland, **445–461**
CT imaging, cross-sectional, of thyroid gland, 449–450
    of parathyroid glands, 543, 544–545
CT scan, multislice, and recurrent thyroid cancer, 519
Cysts, parathyroid, 538, 539, 542, 547

E

Elastography, of thyroid nodules, 465
Esophageal diverticulum, 484, 487

F

Fat, retro-ocular, in Graves disease, 531, 533
Fine needle aspiration, of thyroid nodules, 476–477, 498–499
    ultrasound-guided, to assess metastatic disease, 484–485
Fluorine 18 fluorodeoxyglucose PET, in recurrent thyroid cancer, 520, 523–524
Follicular neoplasms, 469, 470
Follicular thyroid carcinoma, 453
    clinical presentation of, 496
    incidence of, 496
    pathology of, 496
    prognosis in, 496

G

Gamma camera, for radioiodine imaging, 505, 506
Goiter, cancer in, 454, 455
    diffuse, imaging and treatment of, 507–508
    multinodular, euthyroid, 510
        hyperthyroidism in, 510
    thyroid, 450–451
Granulomas, foreign body, 484, 486
Graves disease. See also *Thyroid ophthalmopathy*.
    classification of eye changes in, 529
    clinical features of, 528–530
    corneal involvement in, 530
    diagnosis of, imaging in, 530
    differential diagnosis of, 531–532, 534
    extraocular muscle involvement in, 529–530
    imaging and treatment of, 507, 508
    imaging in, 530–531
    incidence of, 527
    names used for, 527
    optic nerve compression in, 531, 533
    orbital decompression in, 534, 535
    pathology and pathophysiology of, 527–528
    proptosis in, 529
    retro-ocular fat expansion in, 531, 533
    retro-ocular fat infiltration in, 531, 533
    soft tissue involvement in, 529
    treatment of, 532–535
    vision loss in, 530
    Werner NO SPECS classification of, 529
    with muscle involvement, 530–531, 532, 534

H

Hashimoto thyroiditis, 467, 468
Hürthle-cell carcinoma, 469, 470
    pathology of, 496–497
Hyperparathyroidism, 551
    calcimimetics in, 557
    epidemiology of, 551–552
    history and physical examination in, 552–553
    primary, 537
    secondary, 537
    surgery in. See *Parathyroidectomy*.
    tertiary, 537
Hyperthyroidism, evaluation of, 447
    imaging and treatment of, 507
    in multinodular goiter, 510
Hypothyroidism, 447
    imaging and treatment of, 508

Index

I

Incidentalomas, thyroid, 513, 514
Insular thyroid carcinoma, pathology of, 496–497
Iodine, radioactive, 505
Iodine-124 whole-body PET imaging, in non-iodine avid thyroid disease, 513, 514
Isotopes, common, radiation-absorbed dose of, 507
  for radioiodine imaging and treatment of thyroid disorders, 506–507

L

Laryngopharyngeal surgery, thyroid surgery and, 501
Larynx and trachea, invasion of thyroid cancer into, surgical management of, 522
Lymph nodes, cervical. See *Cervical lymph node(s).*
  ultrasound for preoperative evaluation of, 485–486
Lymphadenopathy, local invasion of thyroid nodules and, 469, 476
Lymphoma, of thyroid, pathology of, 498
  primary, of thyroid, 454, 471

M

Medullary thyroid carcinoma, 453–454, 470
  clinical presentation of, 497
  encapsulation of, 497
  pathology of, 497
  polypeptide hormones secreted by, 497
MR imaging, cross-sectional, of thyroid gland, 450
  of parathyroid glands, 545–548
Multiple endocrine neoplasia, 538

N

Neck, anatomy of, 493–494
  compartments of, 493
Neoplasms, malignant, of thyroid gland, 451–458
  thyroid, 467–468
Neuromas, post-thyroidectomy, 484, 486
Nuclear medicine techniques, for parathyroid imaging, 543–544
Nuclear scintigraphy, of thyroid gland, 448–449

O

Ophthalmopathy, thyroid, 447
Optic nerve compression, in Graves disease, 531, 533
Orbital decompression, in Graves disease, 534, 535

P

Papillary thyroid carcinoma, 452–453
  as multifocal disease, 495
  extrathyroidal extension of, 496
  in metastatic colon cancer, 513, 514
  pathology of, 494–496
  prognosis in, 496
  recurrent, 457–458
  variants of, 494
  vascularity in, 475
Parathyomatosis, 538–539, 541
Parathyroid adenoma, 537, 538, 542, 547, 554
  ectopic, 544
Parathyroid carcinoma, 538, 540
Parathyroid cysts, 538, 539, 542, 547
Parathyroid gland(s), 493
  anatomy of, 537
  CT of, interpretation of, 545
    pitfalls of, 545, 546
    technique of, 544
  embryology of, 537, 552
  imaging of, 539–548
  MR imaging of, interpretation of, 545–548
    pitfalls of, 548
    technique of, 545
  nuclear medicine imaging of, interpretation of, 543–544
    pitfalls of, 544
    technique of, 543
  operative anatomy of, 554–555
  pathology of, 537–539
  ultrasound of, interpretation of, 540–541, 542
    pitfalls of, 541–543
    technique of, 539–540, 542
Parathyroid hormone, secretion of, 551
Parathyroid imaging, **537–549**
Parathyroid surgery, what radiologists need to know, **551–558**
Parathyroidectomy, indications for, 552, 553
  operative assistance techniques in, 555–556
  operative considerations for, 555
  postoperative considerations for, 556–557
  preoperative evaluation for, 553–554
  reoperative setting for, 556
Pharyngoesophageal diverticulum, 484, 487
Positron emission tomography, fluorine 18 fluorodeoxyglucose, in recurrent thyroid cancer, 520, 523–524
  iodine-124 whole-body, in non-iodine avid thyroid disease, 513, 514

R

Radiation, external beam, in recurrent thyroid cancer, 523
Radioiodine imaging, and treatment in thyroid disorders, **505–515**
  instrumentation for, 505, 506
  isotopes for, 506–507

patient preparation for, 505–506
and treatment of differentiated thyroid cancer, 511–512
Radiologist(s), need to know about parathyroid surgery, **551–558**
need to know of surgical approaches to thyroid cancer, **491–504**

S

Single photon emission computed tomography, of parathyroid glands, 543
Sonographic imaging, of cervical lymph nodes, in thyroid cancer, **479–489**
  technique of, 480
Squamous cell carcinoma, of thyroid, 454

T

Thyroglobulin, rising, imaging of treated thyroid gland with, 457–458
Thyroglobulin levels, serum, and recurrent thyroid cancer, 518–519
Thyroglossal duct cysts, and carcinoma, 458–459
Thyroid, anatomy of, 463–465, 492–493
  arterial supply to, 492
  benign adenomas of, 451
  cross-section imaging of, **445–461**
  development and anatomy of, 445–446
  disease of, clinical manifestations of, 447–448
    non-iodine avid, iodine-124 whole-body PET imaging in, 513, 514
  disorders of, radioiodine imaging and treatment in, **505–515**
  embryology of, 492
  endocrinology of, 446–447
  imaging of, 448–450
    radionuclides used in, 448
  lymphatics of, 492–493
  malignant neoplasms of, 451–458
  mass of, workup of, management algorithm for, 499
  metastatic disease of, 454, 469, 471–472
  midline ectopic masses of, sites of, 492
  nerves of, 493
  nodular diseases of, 450
  scanning of, technique of, 463–465
  surgery of, and laryngopharyngeal surgery, 501
    extended, 500–501
    extent of, pathologic findings influencing, 500
    for locally advanced thyroid cancer, 501–502
    in cancer invasionr into surrounding structures, 501
    neck dissection in, extent of, 501
    prognostic factors and, 500
    risk group analysis and, 500
    vascular anatomy and, 500
  treated, imaging of, with rising thyroglobulin, 457–458
Thyroid cancer, cervical lymph nodes in, sonographic imaging of, **479–489**
  differentiated, follow-up of, 512
    radioiodine imaging and treatment of, 511–512
    risk of recurrence of, 518, 519
  differentiated lymph node metastases in, 485
  epidemiology of, 491–492
  etiology of, 491
  in low-risk patients, radiodine treatment of, 512
  intermediate- and high-risk, follow-up after treatment of, 512–514
    initial presentation of, 512
  locally advanced, thyroid surgery for, 501–502
  pathology of, 494, 496
  pattern of spread of, 484
  radiologist in evaluation of, 454–457
  recurrent, central compartment in, surgical management of, 521
    cervical ultrasound to diagnose, 519
    decreased survival following, and risk factors for, 518
    diagnosis of, 518–520
    external beam radiation in, 523
    fluorine 18 fluorodeoxyglucose PET in, 520, 523–524
    imaging for detection of, 520
    laryngotracheal invasion in, surgical management of, 522
    long-term survival and, 517
    multislice CT scan and, 519
    reoperation in, risk of, 521–522
    risk factors for, 517–518
    serum thyroglobulin levels and, 518–519
    surgical management of, **517–525**
    thyroid bed in, surgical management of, 521
    thyroid remnant in, surgical management of, 521
    well-differentiated, treatment of, 520–523
    whole-body iodine 131 uptake scan of, 519
  staging of, 494, 495
    and risk management in, 510–511
  surgical approaches to, what radiologist needs to know, **491–504**
Thyroid disease, extrathyroidal manifestations of, thyroid ophthalmopathy in, **527–536**
Thyroid disorders, benign, imaging and treatment of, 507–510
Thyroid goiter, 450–451
Thyroid incidentalomas, 513, 514
Thyroid neoplasms, 467–468
Thyroid nodules, calcifications of, 474
  calculation of volume of, 464
  cancerous, 451
  cystic, and ring-down artifact, 474–475

Thyroid (*continued*)
  echogeniciy of, 474
  elastrography of, 465
  evaluation of, 509–510
    and management of, 498–499
  fine needle aspiration of, 476–477, 498–499
  growth of, 474
  hyperplastic, 466–467
    eggshell calcification of, 468
  imaging of, preoperative, 499
    sonographic technologies in, 464–465
  laboratory evaluation of, 498
  local invasion of, and lymphadenopathy, 469, 476
  metastasis to, 471–472
  multivariate analyses of, 476
  1 cm or larger diameter, management of, 476
  prevalence of, 463
  shape and margins of, 469, 475, 476
  size and multiplicity of, 472–474
  solitary, hyperfunctioning, 509–510
    hypofunctioning, 510
  sonographic features of, 472–476
  types of, 465–466
  ultrasound of, **463–478**
  vascularity of, 475
Thyroid ophthalmopathy, 447
  as extrathyroidal manifestation of thyroid disease, **527–536**

Thyroidectomy bed, normal, 484, 486
  recurrent thyroid cancer in, 484, 485, 486
    mimics of, 484, 486, 487
Thyroiditis, chronic, imaging and treatment of, 508
  subacute and silent, hypothyroidism in, 508
    imaging and treatment of, 507–508
    thyrotoxicosis in, 507
Thyrotoxicosis, 447
  associated with hyperthyroidism, 447
  in thyroiditis, 507

U

Ultrasound, cervical, to diagnose recurrent thyroid cancer, 519
  of parathyroid glands, 539–543
  of thyroid gland, 449
  of thyroid nodules, **463–478**
  preoperative lymph node evaluation using, 485–486
Ultrasound-guided fine needle aspiration, to assess metastatic disease, 484–485

V

Vision loss, in Graves disease, 530

Moving?

Make sure your subscription moves with you!

To notify us of your new address, find your **Clinics Account Number** (located on your mailing label above your name), and contact customer service at:

E-mail: elspcs@elsevier.com

800-654-2452 (subscribers in the U.S. & Canada)
1-407-563-6020 (subscribers outside of the U.S. & Canada)

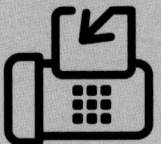

Fax number: 407-363-9661

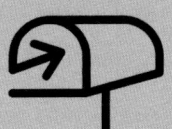

Elsevier Periodicals Customer Service
6277 Sea Harbor Drive
Orlando, FL 32887-4800

*To ensure uninterrupted delivery of your subscription, please notify us at least 4 weeks in advance of move.

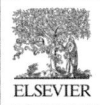